# GOOD PRACTICE *to* THRIVING PRACTICE

## SECRETS FROM SOME OF AMERICA'S BUSIEST DENTAL PROFESSIONALS AND HOW THEY ACHIEVED MASSIVE PRACTICE GROWTH DURING A SLOW ECONOMY

## MICHAEL HILL

*To my wife and sons-*
*dream, strive, and thrive!*

# Contents

# Your Always Busy Dental Practice

It turns out owning a dental practice is not all roses and rainbows. In fact, a lot of dentists that I know personally are struggling to make ends meet.

After all those years of study and dedication, it is a blow to your ego to realize just how much of a challenge owning a business is going to be in this economy.

But there it is—you can either accept the challenge or become buried by dentists in your area that have.

They will take your clients, and they will take your income. This is a competitive landscape we are dealing with here. There is no longer any safety in the concept of the "family" dentist. Those days are gone!

I have watched firsthand the terrible struggle of many dental offices. Some of my dentist friends have been forced to sell their practices, some have just closed their doors, and others, who manage to remain open, simply putter along with poor performing practices. They rarely meet their production goals and their team turnover is very high. They are in desperate need of better structuring, systems, and marketing.

I work with more than 100 dental offices in several different states. I have seen the damage that can be inflicted when dentists refuse or simply do not have the skill set to effectively take on the operational functions necessary to build and maintain a successful dental practice.

Within two blocks of my office, there are four dentists. One is always busy and constantly on the go. The other has good months and bad ones. The last two, well…they drag their feet. They are always talking about the problem but never seem to find any solutions.

My reality is that my business is utterly dependent upon the success of dentists. I decided to write this book because I simply had too many instances of watching my dental clients and friends throw good money after bad as they tried to use one or two advertising tactics to "turn around" their practice. That style or brand of management results in a long and expensive road to practice mediocrity.

On the other hand, there is a well-traveled path for building a thriving practice. It is well documented, totally researched, and easily observed, and it is contained within the pages of this book.

Three years in the making, this guide to a thriving practice contains contributions from more than 60 dentists, office managers, treatment planners, consultants, practice sales agents, dental lab owners, practice financing companies, and researchers.

Collectively, these individuals work with both struggling practices and thriving practices. With their help, we have identified 20 of the top disciplines and strategies that thriving practices have in common.

Dentists with thriving practices have paved the way. They have already endured the financial pain of trial and error. The ground work is laid, and the path to a massively successful dental practice is illuminated.

Now you can benefit from these experiences by following these same amazing strategies that have given thriving practices and their teams such dynamic direction and success.

*Section*

# 01

# Time For Your
# Sweet Tooth
*(Self-Development
Strategy)*

## chapter 1

# The Altitude of Your Personal Attitude

"Attitude is a little thing that makes
a big difference."
WINSTON CHURCHILL

What is your attitude like towards the work that you do every day? Towards your patients and employees? Could it be better? I would argue that it can be.

My personal attitude was not something that I thought about very often until I realized what a huge impact it had on my business and my life.

Defined, your attitude is a "learned tendency to evaluate things in a certain way."[1] That means everything from the people in your life to the events, issues, and objects that affect you will result in either a positive or negative attitude.

Have you ever heard that saying "your attitude determines your altitude"? It means that the WAY that you approach things essentially determines if they will be successful or not.

---

1    Kendra, Cherry, How Attitudes Form, Change and Shape Our Behavior, http://psychology.about.com/od/socialpsychology/a/attitudes.htm

It is a powerful concept and one that too many dentists prefer to ignore. Who cares what your attitude is about your work, right? It is work! Well, the world cares.

There are three aspects involved in determining your attitude: emotions, cognitive responses, and behavior. They work together to create your chosen attitude.

Notice that I say chosen because attitude is a choice. Your emotions dictate how you feel about something, your thoughts and beliefs shape how you think about it, and then your behavior is driven by those emotions and thoughts.

Your attitude is a collection of your life experiences and learned behaviors as a child. It is the first thing you need to change if you are intent on building a solid dental practice.

- The right attitude energizes and motivates you. It puts that passion that you once had for your patients and their problems in your heart.

- A positive attitude at work is infectious—if you are fiercely positive about your practice, your employees will feel the same way. Walk around gloomy all day, and all hope will be lost!

- Being a dentist with the right attitude means lower stress levels and increased endorphins in your brain.[2] Happiness is always close by when you focus on having the right attitude about things.

- According to WorldHealth.net,[3] having a positive attitude promotes wellbeing and health, which means that the more you practice it, the better you feel.

---

2    Maria Osnowitz, Endorphins = Happy = Positive, Dr Oz Show, http://www. doctoroz.com/blog/maria-osnowitz/endorphins-happy-positive

3    Positive Attitude Promotes Well-Being, http://www.worldhealth.net/news/ positive-attitude-promotes-well-being/

There you go. Medical science supports the theory that the right attitude in fact DOES determine your altitude in life. There are volumes of research that have been done on attitude and how mentally strong people succeed in business.

Call me old fashioned, but having read a lot of this research and practiced it in person—to great effect—I have to say this method works. Thinking negative things all the time is soul destroying—and it does not help you one bit.

So your personal attitude matters in more ways than you previously believed. The only remaining thing to do is employ some of these incredible attitude-changing habits.

Thriving dentists have an attitude that puts patients at ease, instills trust and loyalty in the minds of your employees, and helps you build a better dental practice.

One of my thriving clients sends me no less than 70 cases every month. He is a remarkably positive human being. Every time I get off the phone with him I feel better about myself. Imagine how his patients feel. His positive, humble, and caring disposition has an incredibly positive impact on his practice.

- **Affirmations or short phrases repeated out loud several times a day** have been proven by science[4] to help reprogram subconscious thought. Using them will go a long way in forcing psychological change so that you can be more positive in life.

- **Practice motivating yourself to action** by being enthusiastic about important things and focusing your energy on being someone who is always willing to help.

- **Visualize who you want to be and where you want to be to make it come true.** Performance psychology

---

4    Self-Affirmation Enhances Performance Makes Us Receptive To Our Mistakes, https://www.psychologicalscience.org/index.php/news/releases/self-affirmation-enhances-performance-makes-us-receptive-to-our-mistakes.html

indicates that the best surgeons in the world use these techniques to enhance skill and focus.

- **Fix that negative self-talk.** Our inner voice can be a real jerk sometimes. Words are powerful; make sure that the ones you use in your mind are gentle, positive, and encouraging.

- **Motivate yourself by lightening up.** Humor is a great tool for building bridges, and you can use it to train yourself to be more positive about your life and your practice.

- **Exercise is a good way to stay energized and motivated,** which is exactly what you are going to need during this process of rebuilding your practice.

## chapter 2

# Embracing Your Business Vision

*"A leader's role is to raise people's aspirations for what they can become and to release their energies so they will try to get there."*

DAVID GERGEN

A large part of self-development is accepting responsibility for your not-so-perfect planning skills. I had to, and I believe it is something that most dentists have to face as well.

Your dental practice was built on a vision that you had for it. Did you ever write this vision down? Did you ever develop the vision strategy to its fullest potential?

A squeaky clean business vision is all about creating goals and objectives for your practice that will give it the direction that it needs to grow. Without growth, your practice will become stagnant. There is no point investing in a stagnant practice.

Every—not almost every, but EVERY—thriving dental practice I work with has a dentist who has written down his precise vision and plan for his dental practice. It makes sense too. How can you lead your team to a goal that is not well defined? How can your team perform at a level that meets your expectations when they do not have a clear idea of what your expectations really are?

Employee retention will plummet, and patients will be similarly unimpressed by your practice's progress. It matters to everyone that you grow, update, and expand.

That is why you need to actively embrace your business vision. That means sitting down and creating a new vision statement so that you can realign your practice with your goals and objectives for the future.

Vision statements can be broken into short-term and long-term statements,5 if you want to get specific. Thriving dentists get as specific as possible.

This element of your business infrastructure must not be confused with your mission statement in your business plan. The two focus on slightly different areas.

Whether you have been in dentistry for five years or 20, preparing your new vision statement has far-reaching benefits for your practice, so do not take it for granted.

At this point, I want you to consider creating two kinds of vision statement: your personal vision statement and your business vision statement.

Creating the two of these together will ensure that you are able to keep them aligned and working in conjunction for your ultimate benefit.

- Your personal mission statement details the goals and objectives that you have for your life or career in the long term.

- Your business mission statement outlines the goals and objectives that you have for your practice in the short and long term.

---

5   Elaine, Hom, What Is a Vision Statement?, http://www.businessnewsdaily. com/3882-vision-statement.html

Bain and Company[6] conducted an interesting study that proved organizations that have a clearly defined vision statement that is aligned with a strategic plan outperform companies that do not have one.

- Vision statements also attract the right kind of employee and help you retain the people that run your business.

- Vision statements are key in promoting business culture and improving productivity in your practice. It should define your desired future state and the time it will take to get there.

- This vision will help communicate to your patients what you are all about, what makes you different, and why they should be loyal to your brand.

Many practices place their vision statement on a wall where it can motivate their staff and generate positive feedback from their patients. Here is how you should create yours.

- Sit down and grab a piece of paper or open your laptop. A vision statement should spell out the high level goals for your practice.

- What do you want your practice to be? Think about growth, values, employees, contributions to society, and your place in your community.

- Your vision statement will drive the rest of your strategy for your dental practice. It is a crucial element and needs to be aligned with your personal goals.

- Consider your patients, your employees, and your practice when drafting your statement—this is the success "triangle" to target.[7]

6    Christopher Bart, A Model Of The Impact of Mission Statements on Firm Performance, http://www.emeraldinsight.com/journals. htm?articleid=865190&show=pdf

7    Wade Mayfield, 3 Key Steps To Creating an Effective Vision Statement, http:// www.hvacrbusiness.com/vision-statement.html

According to James Collins of the Harvard Business review,[8] articulating a clear vision for your practice involves focusing on your core ideology and your envisioned future.

Your core ideology will involve your practice's values and purpose, while your envisioned future will contain your 10–30 year big, hairy, audacious goals and a vivid description of them.

By ticking all the boxes with your vision statement, your patients should understand who you are and where you are going. They are more likely to be loyal to you and will say something if you depart from your vision.

Being publicly open about your vision means that accountability is valued at your practice. Not only will commitments be met, but you are saying to your patients that they can expect bigger and better things from you in the future.

---

8    James Collins, Building Your Company's Vision, http://hbr.org/1996/09/building-your-companys-vision/ar/1

chapter 3

# The Psychology of Personal Branding

*"Your premium brand had better be delivering something special, or it's not going to get the business."*

WARREN BUFFETT

Your practice has a brand, and that brand is constantly broadcasting a message to your patients, employees, and colleagues. What does yours say? Knowing how to create a relatable brand image is not just something that rock star advertising agencies do. You are selling a service, and that service needs to be ultra-clear in the minds of your repeat patients.

Defined, a personal brand is a "powerful, clear, positive idea that comes to mind whenever other people think of you."[9]

Being a dentist, your personal brand is very closely associated with your practice's brand. In fact, you could say that the two are intimately aligned.

---

9    Peter Montoya, The Brand Called You, http://www.petermontoya.com/pdfs/tbcy-chapter1.pdf

Your personal brand is linked with your vision statements, so make sure that the one works with the other. At the end of the day, this is what influences your patients' decisions.

A professional alter ego is something that you need to build if you are going to be the preferable choice among competitors in your area.

There is some real psychology involved in this process that I will speak about here. When you know how to project an image, you know how to communicate a story.

Unofficially, personal branding is a method of communicating your core self to your target market, in this case, your patients.

Everything from your personal goals, talents, values, and fascinations makes you a unique individual. When you can communicate this effectively, you will not only attract the right employees but the right patients to your practice.

- According to Psychcentral,[10] a brand always stands for something. What do you stand for? If you can figure this out, you will excel at personal branding.

- A strong personal brand allows you to grow your network of contacts and important people much faster than normal.

- It acts like a magnet, attracting opportunities to you from employees, other practices, health organizations, and patients.

- It establishes you as a powerfully credible individual who is trustworthy, reliable, and willing to go the extra mile to conduct good business.

- It does a lot for your online presence and makes the transition from real world promotion[11] to digital promotion a snap. This is insanely important.

10  Lisa Miles, Self-Image, Identity and The Tools of Personal Branding, http://psychcentral.com/blog/archives/2013/07/10/self-image-identity-the-tools-of-personal-branding/

11  Roxanne Hori, The Importance of Managing Your Personal Brand, http://www.businessweek.com/articles/2013-11-22/the-importance-of-managing-your-personal-brand

- It attaches a bold personality to your brand that will drive all future business processes and success in your niche.

When you take some time to develop your personal brand, it will communicate to your patients that you are a fair, level-headed, compassionate, kind, and endlessly detail-orientated dentist who towers over others in your area.

The goal is always to project the image that you are the leader in your field and your community—and as such, you know what your patients need.

As you begin to establish your brand, you must take into account the demographics of your local market. Trying to create an image as a super high end dental spa in a predominantly lower income community is a disconnected strategy.

**ALISSA BLOUIN**

The Marketing Director at Keystone Dental Arts, reinforces this strategy:

*"Many wonderful dentists with great reputations do NOT have 'Saks Fifth Avenue' level practices, and much of their clientele would not respond well to that type of office/strategy; they would feel that they were overpaying for luxury that they do not want/need, especially if such an office has discount offices and other hungry heavily marketed competition around the corner."*

Create a brand that is consistent with your personal goals but that can also be effective within the market you serve. An effective and distinct brand that has a message that resonates with your target patient base will deliver substantial growth for your practice.

**AMOL NIRGUDKAR**

Author of *Profitable Niches in General Dentistry*
and founder of Dentist Profit Systems LLC
added this thought:

*"You just need to cater to your local demographic better than your competition. Once the value proposition is instilled in the mind of the consumer, they will pay more and come to you. Actually, it is very easy to compete with Aspen or Coast or any of the big companies (in our market). You just have to tell your story right."*

So how do you stand out from your competing practices in a way that will have the most impact on your bottom line? Follow these tactics.

- All branding is based on authenticity, so be truthful when putting together your personal brand.

- What is it that makes you different? What is your super power? What can you do that is absolutely better than anyone else you know? Write it down.

- What do people tend to come to you for? Can you identify why they trust you with this particular procedure or process?

- What guiding principles allow you to operate in your practice? List your core values and why you believe that they are important.

- What is it that you get the most praise and compliments for? People are a reliable feedback mechanism—it would suit you to institute some big data strategy to help you develop a stronger personal brand.

- How do you do what you do? Document any unique processes, procedures, or service-level practices that make you different and better.

- Where do your passions lie? Passion drives progress, and when you are upfront about your passion, people respond in a positive manner.

- Pick one prominent thing that you want to be known for,[12] and people will flock to you for it. Everyone cannot be good at everything. Identify where your strengths lie, and build them into your very own personal brand.

---

12  Siimon Reynolds, How You Can Build a Great Personal Brand, http://www.forbes. com/sites/siimonreynolds/2014/02/06/how-you-can-build-a-great-personal-brand/

chapter 4

# Connecting With Patient X

*"Communication—the human connection—is the key to personal and career success."*

PAUL J. MEYER

E ngaging with patients is perhaps the single most important method of instilling faith in your practices and dental practice.

While it is crucial to perform procedures correctly, accurately, and with the greatest care, it all means nothing if it is done with a poor attitude or one that makes the patient uncomfortable and unwilling to return.

Time and time again a good experience at the dentist office is worth a thousand dollar investment in advertising to find new patients.

Your sole goal should be to get existing patients to return and to do it with a smile on their faces. That means learning how to connect with patient X. You need to build rapport quickly.

**ALEX NOTTINGHAM,** MBA, JD

Founder, and CEO of All Star Dental Academy,
puts it this way:

*"Rapport isn't about 'being best friends' with patients. It means creating a comfortable 'state' where conversation runs smoothly, the experience is enjoyable, and the results meet our, and importantly, the patient's expectations. There's a lot more to building rapport and trust than making an initial good impression and connection with someone, but it's a critical start. And making a connection with someone makes them more comfortable sharing with you their needs and desires."*

Patient X is the worst kind of patient. They hate dentists,[13] and they recoil at your touch. Every procedure is preceded by anxiety, anger, fear, and ill feelings. If you can connect with this patient, then serving others will be easy.

One of the most important things you can do as a dentist is to walk your patients through what needs to happen and why—AND what is happening and why. Long needles full of burning liquid and scary drilling noises are how most people view dentists.

If you can educate your patients and focus on helping them understand their treatment options and your methods of performing them, closer relationships will result.

I think that you will find a large percentage of your "never to return" patients are a direct result of poor doctor–patient experiences. That can be eliminated from your practice.

Many of my dentist clients focus on finding out exactly

---

13 Thursday Troubleshooter: Dental Patient Won't Complete Medical Forms, http://www.dentistryiq.com/articles/2013/12/thursday-troubleshooter1.html

what their patients need from them as opposed to telling their patients what they need—it helps a lot. You can do this by collecting data from various touch points in your practice's business model. Places like online, surveys, in-practice polls, and personal interviews are valuable.

- According to BMC Health Services Research,14 patients worry about new techniques, preventative measures, and things going wrong with old procedures.
- Fred Joyal of 1800dentist[15] says that it is because your practice does not offer what they want, and often this means the latest, least intrusive treatments.
- Patients have also made it clear on numerous occasions that they have no idea what a dentist does when they are inside your mouth. Explain it to them!
- Patients see cost as a stumbling block and often cannot make sense of why some treatments are so expensive. This needs to be transparent!
- Many patients cannot tolerate the guilt they feel when they delay cleanings or appointments, and this is further exacerbated by "reminders."

As you can see, there may be more than one patient connection problem at work in your practice right now. They all add up to create a set of very clear reasons why you should invest more of your time into your personal relationships with your patients.

There is a strong need for better patient connection and education in your practice. You can strengthen your current practices by instituting these changes:

---

14  Alexandra, Sbaraini, Experiences of Dental Care: What Do Patients Value?, http://www.biomedcentral.com/1472-6963/12/177

15  7 Real-Life Reasons Why Patients Leave, http://www.1800dentist.com/7-reallife-reasons-your-patients-leave/

- Create an education strategy involving patient-centric knowledge in print, online, and in direct communication. Content and conversation combined are great!

- Focus on creating content for your practice that spells out in detail what your patient can expect from certain procedures and what to look for if something goes wrong.

- A small LCD screen above your dentist's chair or a radio can do wonders for a nervous, anxious patient. It lowers their cortisol levels,[16] using distraction as a stress reduction technique.

- Practice using the right supportive language in your practice so that you can gently guide your patient through the procedure without alarm.

- Be aware that patients want to be told what their treatment options are and what you will be doing to them. Spend a good amount of time pre-process explaining this!

- Build a knowledge resource on your website or blog and encourage patients to visit you there with valid questions.

- Get to know your patients! Behave as if you intend on seeing them again in the future. Remember their name, greet them with a smile, and learn about their family and friends.

If you take some time to sit down and outline the various patient X techniques that you will use in your practice, implementation will be easier. Then you can actively measure your progress and see if the improved connections are boosting your business.

---

16  Robert McMaster, Practical Considerations For Treating The Anxious Dental Patient, http://www.oralhealthgroup.com/news/practical-considerations-for-treating-the-anxious-dental-patient/1000880281/?&er=NA

## chapter 5

# The Doctor Is In: Self-Examination and Pacing

"Adopt the pace of nature:
her secret is patience."

RALPH WALDO EMERSON

Your patients have needs, and you are the main person who is responding to those needs. As a result, you have also become the key human asset in your practice.

The ramifications of this are fairly straightforward—if you overwork yourself, your patient care quality will plummet. If you try to rush through patient care, you will never attain the standard you are looking to achieve.

Learning how to pace yourself through self-examination is instrumental in running a successful dental practice. It begins with you admitting that your methods are not perfect.

For every successful dentist visit, there are several others that have failed—and this can be chalked up to your ability to maintain your own standards.

Even the most thriving dentists have bad days, and I know plenty of dentists that are not "people" orientated. But the key lesson here is that pacing improves service delivery, and you are in charge of it.

Think about the average visitation process—patients come in when something is wrong to get it fixed or to have a cleaning. They often leave things until the last moment.

To prepare for this common eventuality and make it a patient-centric experience, you will need to build in levels of patient care based on pacing structures.

A patient needs to be told in detail what their diagnosis is and what their treatment options are. They need to understand what will happen during each procedure, how much it will cost, and what the post-treatment recovery will entail.

In some cases, the need for preparation and time management is overlooked because the dentist involved needs to see more patients than time allows.

While this may seem to solve the initial financial pressure, it works out in the long term against your business interests. Here are some reasons why you need to refocus your attention on yourself and on managing your time better.

- Evidence-based clinical practice[17] will help you identify where you need to spend more of your time. Modern technologies and software can also streamline your day.

- Thinking of new ways to improve preventative measures in your patients will not diminish from your bottom line— quite the opposite.

- A smart dentist would institute the help of an app or software to monitor their patients' oral health. With a direct line to you, questions can be answered, genuine service can be

---

17  Dental Practice-Based Research To Improve Oral Health and To Support The Adoption of Evidence-Based Clinical Practice, http://www.nidcr.nih.gov/ GrantsAndFunding/See_Funding_Opportunities_Sorted_By/ConceptClearance/ CurrentCC/PracticeBasedResearch.htm

given, and patients will always come to you when they need something done.

- Look after yourself by learning more about your habits, strengths, and weaknesses. Focus on making time for business, family and fun so that you are a balanced person and a healthy individual.

- Time saving resources like online websites, apps, or flowcharts of your patient procedures will go a long way in freeing up more of your precious time.

- When you schedule clients, make sure that you take breaks, have lunch, and stop working at reasonable hours so that you can always provide the highest level of service excellence.

Self-examination and getting to know who you are and how you behave goes a long way in helping you manage your time. If you are going to improve your patient care, you must become one of the most important people in your practice. In order to achieve this, integrate the following into your personal development plan:

- *Learn to delegate.* Thriving dentists have a laser focus on their patients and the complete patient experience. Everything else, like admin, marketing, patient orientation, making crowns on digital machines, and more, can go to other employees. You diminish your value to your practice and take away precious time with your patients if you cannot master delegation.

- *Use evidence-based clinical practice[18] to find out where you waste your time.* Measure your processes, procedures, and work flows. Unearth the parts of your business that are draining all your time away.

---

18  Preparation and Time Management, American Dental Association, http://www.ada.org/5439.aspx

- *Focus on monthly scheduling, and tier it down.* Establish thresholds so that if you become "overloaded," your system kicks in and you have to consider hiring another dentist for your practice.

- *Pacing means having a schedule that is properly managed* with the help of modern software and technologies like tablets, apps, and mobile systems.

- *Make yourself accountable to someone in your practice*, and ask them to help you meet your pacing goals.

If you can achieve these goals, you will find that managing your dental practice becomes a whole lot easier—because you have the energy to do it! Not only that, but your patients will have better experiences, which means more repeat visits.

# **Practice Teething Problems**
## ***(Treatment Strategy)***

## chapter 6

# The Science of Practice Aesthetics: First Impressions Last

"It is only at the first encounter that a face makes its full impression on us."

ARTHUR SCHOPENHAUER

Y ou have reached section two, where you will discover a few important tactics to use in your overall treatment strategy.

There is a real science involved when working with what a dental practice "looks like." In the old days you used to walk into a stark white, slightly aging office block, surrounded by the smell of chemicals and the melody of drills buzzing in the background.

I cannot stress enough the importance of having a welcoming environment. Your patient experience begins the very moment they set foot into your practice.

What your practice looks like and FEELS like will be the first impression they will get of you. If your practice looks shoddy, but they have a good experience, they will still have that doubt about you because of your poor image.

The only way to fix this is to understand that looks matter to people. A patient wants to enter a clean, warm, and safe environment that is exceedingly professional, organized, and neat. If your offices are not modern, what are the chances that your treatments will be?

You have to learn about the power of first impressions and how they impact your patient services. Dentists of thriving dental practices consider every visit from a repeat patient an opportunity to make another "first impression" happen.

Everything is based on first impressions these days, from the rise of online media to the kind of cake that you buy at the bakery. People want things to look right.

So what contributes to the aesthetics of a dentist practice? People, processes, and—of course—the overall appearance of your rooms. These are critical because:

- Unwelcoming staff can make even the most modern dental practice feel like a harsh environment. If your patient does not feel like they belong, they will not come back. The busiest dental practices I work with have unbelievably friendly and thoughtful office staff. Conversely, most of our slowest clients have staff that are generally cool, short, distracted, and uninterested. You may like your team, but that is because you have taken the time to get to know them and the goodness within them that is not always immediately apparent. Your patients must have an immediately positive experience. They need to like your team within seconds of meeting them. Everyone else is keeping you from thriving, and if they do not have that skill set, you need to clean house.

- Overworked staff will leave the patient waiting for too long, giving them the hint that the processes in the business do not allow for quality of service.

- Sitting in old tattered chairs or on outdoor furniture is no way to instill faith in your dental staff. Investing in clean, modern offices with new technology goes a very long way with patients these days.

- Your job is to be the opposite of your patient's worst fear[19]—which is that cold, clinical, and extremely traumatizing dentist visit that horror movies are made of. Warmth, friendly service, and fun are exactly what is required to counteract this image.

- If you want to target word of mouth advertising, make your office and staff profile different. Updating your practice with new paint alone can have a very positive impact on your office as your patients see your attention to detail and growth. Updated lobbies give your team a sense of pride. Your patients will comment on the new décor, and your team will proudly smile while being reminded that they work for a great dentist.

If you are going to go ahead and create that exceptional dentist office experience, then you will need some powerful tactics in your practice arsenal.

- Always smile, greet, and take a moment or two with a patient if you see them outside of your official office. This includes general office areas or outside work. Tell and train your staff to do the same thing.

- Never be too busy for a patient; it makes them feel insignificant. Your goal is to make them feel like they belong, are welcome, and are in safe hands.

- Your exterior and interior aesthetics count, so keep paint jobs clean and technology modern, and never allow old furniture or décor to chase away your patients.

---

19 Survey: What Patients Like About The Dental Office Experience, http://www.dentistryiq.com/articles/2012/12/survey-what-do-patients-like-about-dental-offices.html

- Add therapeutic value to your rooms. Gentle music, televisions, gaming consoles, or play areas for the kids are nice ideas that turn a rigid dental office into a warm office for real people.

- Take care of the extras to enhance your patient experience— lavender towels, VIP parking, modern accents, scented soaps, fresh mouthwash, LCD televisions in each room, and clean, comfortable facilities.

- Leverage the time spent in the waiting room by offering patients a choice of educational videos[20] to watch about dental health. You can also offer them movies, reading material, or music to keep them comfortable.

---

**GIL MORLOCK**

CEO at Universal Healthcare
Practice Solutions, Inc., added this:

*"So what is the secret sauce? The answer is: clearly understanding people, knowing that people need to feel good about their purchases. That's why I own a black SUV in Scottsdale, Arizona, where the average temperature is over one 100. It's not practical, but it makes me feel good to drive that beautiful, black, shiny SUV. Clearly understanding how people think and how we as humans go about making decisions is the foundation to a successful relationship with your dental patients.*

---

20  Renee Knight, Products For an Efficient Dental Practice and Enhanced Patient Experience [Video], http://www.dentalproductsreport.com/dental/article/products-efficient-dental-practice-and-enhanced-patient-experience-video

Draw a road map of every point of contact in your practice. For example: the first call, the first time they see your practice from the road, the first time they walk into your reception area, and so on. Then analyze each point of contact to determine the potentials for a positive experience. Your road map should start way before the initial contact and continue until it comes to a full circle."

## chapter 7

# Quality Consistency and Systematizing Treatment Options

*"Clarity and consistency are not enough: the quest for truth requires humility and effort."*

TARIQ RAMADAN

The next part of your new treatment strategy is going to involve rapidly improving your quality of treatment by systematizing all of your treatment processes.

When someone on Facebook asks for the best dentist in their area, someone in your area should give them your name. Being known for high quality treatments takes efficient planning and strategy.

It is not easy to keep quality consistent when you do not have proper systems in place. A good system will ensure that you establish a tested process that maximizes time, minimizes waste, and works to keep you on track with your quality goals.

The trick with system implementation[21] in your practice is to start by introducing technology that will help you track, analyze,

---

21  Kim Morris, How To Systematize Your Business: The First Step, http:// entrepreneursystems.com/2010/12/how-to-systemize-your-business-the-first-step/

and report on processes and practices that are currently in place. Then you can begin designing and introducing new systems.

A new system, for example, might be how you take a patient through a specific treatment process. The system that is established can be used by anyone and will operate even when you are not around.

In this way, your practice is optimized and relies on best practice systems instead of on individual steam. When you leave processes to chance, that is when quality drops.

I want you to specifically focus on your treatments here. That is your core service profile, and it is the reason why your patients will return.

Learning to minimize treatment problems and maximize treatment success is something that you can include in your overall business operations process. Here are some reasons why systematization of your treatments is essential:

- Your patients will have fewer complications, and they will heal faster because you have ensured that every step of the process works to their advantage.

- In the long term, you will save money because treatment revisions will be unnecessary as they will all have successful outcomes.

- Your patients will never have problems with you, so they will be more inclined to stay loyal to your brand for an indefinite amount of time.

- An excellent reputation in treatment quality will ensure that even though you have a lot of competition, you are still able to come out on top.

- Creating systems or standards of practice will also guarantee that your partners are maintaining the same level of consistent quality22 that you are.

22  Quality Measurement in Dentistry, Dental Quality Alliance, http://www.ada. org/sections/dentalPracticeHub/pdfs/DQA_Guidebook_52913.pdf

Along with systematizing your treatments, you should establish policy that will ensure that your practice never outdates. Working with evidence-based systems is a safe way to make sure that your patients receive an outstanding treatment from you.

There are a variety of ways to systematize your treatment offerings, but really it comes down to the information systems that you have in place.

With quality technology, you can monitor, measure, and test different methods of producing the highest level outcome. Without software, this would be incredibly difficult. That is why when systematizing your treatments, you should focus on the following:

- Evidence-based treatment[23] standards that are part of the intellectual equity of your specific dental practice. Collect data, analyze it, and see what works over time.

- Make sure you stay up to date with the latest technology, treatment options, and machinery so that you can leverage it as it is released.

- The best possible patient experience with the treatment may require manual investigations and feedback to compile real world data.

- Consider that people are different in different communities. Yours may prefer one method of treatment over the other—it is your job to find out what and why.

- Investigate different kinds of business systems and how they can integrate with the testing models that you will set up for systematization.

---

23  Creating Standards For Consistent, High Quality Dental Therapy Education in The United States, http://www.communitycatalyst.org/doc-store/publications/dt-education-report-summary.pdf

Part of your system must include "extras" like machine maintenance processes, repair, data analyzing, report creation, and training of your staff.

To maintain a consistent level of quality in your dental practice takes hard work, but once the system is in place, you will not have to question whether it is the best way to operate.

## chapter 8

# Practice Differentiation and Your USP

*"When positioning a brand, aggressively avoid becoming a 'me too' by assertively being a 'who else?'"*

CRYSTAL BLACK DAVIS

According to the American Dental Association, in 2009 there were 186,084 professionally active dentists in the U.S. At the same time, there were 170,694 active private practitioners. At any given time 90%[24] of these dentists can be found in metropolitan areas.

If you do not live outside of a town, you are probably competing with dozens of other dental practices in your area. That is a fact.

This is why it is highly important at this stage to work differentiation into your treatment strategy. Defining your USP, or unique sales proposition, is exactly what will set you apart in a sea of like-minded competitors.

---

24  KD Nash, Geographic Distribution of Dentists in The United States, http://www.ada.org/sections/professionalResources/pdfs/topics_economic_geo-2011D.pdf

Your USP clearly defines what makes your treatment services valuable to your target demographic. There is a trick you can use here to get the returns that you need.

**DEBORAH BUSH**

Writer and Editor for Dentist Profit Systems LLC says:

*"On top of doing your best to provide exceptional dentistry in an exceptional way and intentionally creating an exceptional online presence, you can observe what your competitors do and develop a niche type or quality of service that is uniquely attractive. That's the way of entrepreneurship."*

All you have to do is find out what makes your closest 10 dental practice competitors unique, nail that down, and then build something better.

There are many ways you can do this as a practice owner, and it is one of the most vital processes involved in reviving your business. The more transparent you can be about what you have to offer your patients, the more chance you have of taking the lion's share of your market.

There is a big difference between guessing and actual research. Evidence-based dentistry is based on the idea that any solid practice can be determined through data and trial and error.

I believe that if you test various unique sales propositions, eventually you will come across one that suits your business culture and your patients' expectations.

Figuring out what differentiates you from the rest is important because:

- Treatment differentiation TELLS your patients something. If, for example, you use the latest modern dental machinery and equipment, this says that you value progressive, less intrusive, more efficient practices.
- Different is often seen as better because it sets you apart from everyone else. This may initially get you the patient traffic that you need.
- A time may come when someone online asks for that dentist in their area that does things differently "from the rest." Your name should come up when they do.
- The actions that you take to help your patients will speak louder than any words or claims. Show people that you are different by BEING something special.

You need that one thing that sets you apart from your competitors, but what is it? A narrow focus will help attract the right kind of patient. Details like office hours,[25] services, payment flexibility, and genuine patient care can all differentiate your practice.

The question now becomes, how? What is the best way to go about quickly and easily discovering what your unique sales proposition might be?

- Create a mastermind group that you can use to bounce your ideas off of. Anyone from your employees, office manager, accountant, and lawyer can be involved.
- Watch for the latest patient trends, feedback, and comments on your online pages, social media, and websites. Try to listen to what people really, really need.
- Redefine your role as a dentist and practice owner. Include patient advisor on this list, and start working towards the

25 Deborah, H, Differentiate Your Dental Practice From The Competition, http://dentainment.com/differentiate-dental-practice/

prevention of problems with their teeth.

- To test different USPs, implement short-term and long-term strategies, then conduct live split testing to determine which ones get the better response.

- Ask! If you do not know what makes you unique, ask the patients that love you already. They may have noticed something you have not.

- Never stop learning. Your unique sales proposition will change over time, and in order to correctly facilitate this process, you need to keep abreast of what is happening in the dental field so that you can adapt and evolve.

With 44% of business owners describing customer retention as critical to achieve growth[26] perhaps you should spend some time developing the concept of your unique sales proposition. A differentiated dental practice today means a better patient retention rate tomorrow.

---

26  Differentiating on Customer Service? What Are The Key Issues?, http://www. customerchampions.co.uk/differentiating-on-customer-service-what-are-the-key-issues/

## chapter 9

# Leveraging Tough-to-Sell Procedures Correctly

*"As a small businessperson, you have no greater leverage than the truth."*

JOHN GREENLEAF WHITTIER

Sometimes, even on your best recommendation, a patient will refuse to have that procedure done to them. Even though this may not even enter your mind, there is a very real chance that you have something to do with their decision. That is why it is important to work out a method of leveraging and selling procedures correctly to your patients to eliminate the chance of this happening.

And even when you do put a system in place, there is still no guarantee that your procedure will sell. You cannot expect to rely on your charm and patient trust to make the sale.

That is why it helps to see the experience from your patient's point of view. They may not have appropriate medical coverage, they may not have cash to pay for the treatment, they may not believe that it is necessary, or they may decide that you are not the dentist to do it.

Any one of these scenarios can arise when you are working closely with patients that require tough-to-sell procedures.

No one likes certain procedures, and when pain is going to be involved, that is essentially what you are selling.

The only way to deal with these instances is to put them in the right context, at the right time, and to have a tested procedure that gets good results in place.

There are many reasons why implementing these sales structures needs to happen. You are not a salesman, first of all, but you are expected to sell certain dental services.

There is an ethical divide that happens here and one that must be addressed. Here are some very good reasons why building a system around procedure sales will help you:

- With access to the Internet, more than your fair share of patients will believe that you are only in it for the money—and that your procedures are nothing more than unnecessary pain and expense.

- A patient may be dealing with personal issues at the time and can therefore not make any important decisions without evidence and guidance. You do not have to pretend when you have data to back up your diagnosis.

- Many cosmetic dental treatments are not necessary, but there are real benefits of having them done. Collect the evidence and lay it out for your patients.

- If your patient feels pushed or forced into the procedure, they will not return to your practice. At the same time, you need to try and sell your services—which is when other types of sales media comes in handy.

- Your patient may want to find out if your pricing is competitive[27] or if they can get it done elsewhere for less. To prevent this, price your procedures fairly and do

---

27 Your Guide To Private Dentistry, Office of Fair Trading, http://www.oft.gov.uk/shared_oft/consumer_leaflets/general/oft660.pdf

a cross section of other dentists in your area. You also need to discover innovative ways to add greater value to a competitive procedure.

How do you go about leveraging these tough-to-sell procedures in a way that will improve sales and that will reduce patient refusal over time? Here is how.

- Divide your treatment pitch into three ideal buyer personas that are based on how "at ease" your patient feels with you. Identify the kind of patient when they visit, and then use the appropriate presentation cycle.

- Create your three types of presentations by conducting research and then testing it live in your practice. Take note of the responses that you get, and document them. Streamline each presentation to suit your ideal patient personas, and use pamphlets as support.

- Package treatments with value added services. Allow patients flexibility in reducing the treatment costs by removing these additional services. Seven thriving dental offices I work with present patients with as many as four different treatment plans. The plans are simple to read and simple to understand, and they clearly list every treatment procedure. Each treatment plan has a different price, and they are defined by both the patients' needs and desires as well as clinical priorities. One of these practices has a treatment coordinator that claims her patient acceptance is 99%. It is a lot different to ask "Which of these treatments would you like to proceed with?" than "Do you want to proceed with the treatment today?"

- Verbal communication is a big part of selling your services. Always put the patient's needs in mind, and offer them a service based on that—not on your need to bring in more sales. Patients can often sense the alternative and will refuse.

- Create a loyalty program[28] that gives the patient direct access to discounts for undesirable procedures at certain times of the year when you know sales will be low.

- Leverage your website and social media, and regularly run competitions to win free treatments. Get feedback and social proof from your winners to try and attract your regular patients the next time they see you online.

---

28  New Patient Loyalty Program Helps Dentists 'Best Recession' Launches At ADA Annual Session, http://www.loyalpatientsinc.com/pdf/Dental%20 Product%20Reports%20October%2020%202008%20Launch%20of%20 Patient%20Program.pdf

# 03

# Grit Your Teeth
# and Hire Them
## *(Employee Strategy)*

## chapter 10

# Populating Your Practice: The Hiring Games

*"If you pick the right people and give them the opportunity to spread their wings and put compensation as a carrier behind it, you almost don't have to manage them".*

JACK WELCH

Section 3 is all about improving your dental practice where it matters most—with your employees. Each and every employee who works for you is part of your brand, and as such, they can either improve its value or decrease its value.

To start with, if your practice is not thriving, it is very possible that you have assembled the wrong team. As you begin to transform your practice by shoring up and upgrading the operational infrastructure as well as act on your new, well-defined vision, you may need to make staff changes quickly.

Your quality of service is directly related to who you decide to hire. Get the right people, and your life will be infinitely easier—get the wrong people, and you are in for a real battle.

You are a dentist, yes, but it is also your job to have final say on your employees. Hiring and firing must be something you are involved in from day 1.

**MARK LIPTON**

Founder of the consulting firm Lipton and Co and chair of the Organizational Change Management program at the Milano Graduate School in New York said:

*"The most important thing to consider (when implementing a new vision or business strategy) is how to communicate it. Not only should people get rewarded when they act in ways thoroughly consistent with the vision, but they should also get punished when their behavior is inconsistent. There's a winnowing process: People who are challenged and motivated by the vision stay and thrive; those who cannot buy into it ultimately leave (or are asked to leave).*

That does not mean that you have to do it all by yourself! By all means, hire a professional, incredibly detail-orientated HR manager to do it for you.

Then set up your hiring systems so that your manager has guidelines to work with and they do not have to guess who you want working for you in your practice.

Once your HR or office manager[29] and employee hiring, management, and firing systems are in place, all you have to do is sign off on the new potential employee.

These may be the hiring games, but you do not have to be on the playing field. Allow your manager to do the legwork for you, and you will get what you need.

Even though you will hire an office manager to take care of your employee hiring processes, you will still have to hire your office manager.

---

29 Hiring an Office Manager For Your Dental Practice, http://www.warschawlearninginstitute.com/showPage.php?pg=HiringanOfficeManagerforYourDentalPractice

This single appointment can make or break your business, so take it very seriously. Your office manager will keep your staff in line and make sure the "daily running" of your practice adheres with your systems, culture, and processes.

Clearly map out the kind of person that you want stepping into your key role as office manager. Make a list of traits, experience, and education, and do not deviate from it.

Make sure that your office manager is constantly on the lookout for great talent. Only hiring when you lose someone is a poor practice—hiring and replacement is an ongoing employee strategy!

If you struggle to identify what you want your employees to be like, create scenarios. These scenarios can become questions that you ask your candidates. A similar answer could reveal a diamond in the rough.

Your office manager will need to be a wizard at multitasking and must have at least three to five years' experience managing a dental or doctor's practice before yours.

Focus on organizational skills, people skills, customer service excellence, and adequate phone skills.[30] These are the building blocks that make a good manager—and they will need to lead by example for your other staff.

So what exactly goes into setting up a good hiring process, and how can you make sure that your office manager adheres to these practice rules? Here is how:

Create a set of strict assessment criteria and media that your office manager can use during your hiring process. This includes advertising templates; behavioral assessments; career, life, and family assessments; and personality checks.

---

30   The Trick To Hiring The Perfect Dental Office Manager For Your Dental Practice, http://www.jointherevo.com/blog/the-trick-to-hiring-the-perfect-front-office-manager-for-your-dental-practice-

Every six months assess your office manager, and point out ways that they can improve while enforcing their key strengths.

Structure your hiring process so that for the first three months your employee is "tested," and if it is a good fit, they will get a permanent employee contract. This eliminates the chance of bad hires affecting your practice too much.

Make sure that your office manager uses modern profiling techniques to research their candidates. This includes documenting their online profile and checking their social media engagement and LinkedIn resume pages.

Create two sets of rules for short-term and long-term hires.[31] Make sure that your employees understand that they need to work to keep their job; it is not a free ride. Standards must be maintained to provide service quality.

I understand that you are busy being a dentist, but these practices and procedures need to be created. If you struggle with them, sit down with your newly hired office manager, and they will help. Get all of your employees to contribute to your hiring process rules.

---

31  John Rossheim, How To Hire Office Staff For a Medical or Dental Practice, http://hiring.monster.com/hr/hr-best-practices/recruiting-hiring-advice/acquiring-job-candidates/how-to-hire-office-staff.aspx

## chapter 11

# The Merits of Human Investment and Ongoing Training

"Leadership and learning are indispensable to each other."

JOHN F. KENNEDY

It is the easiest thing in the world to forget that the people that work for you are also an integral part of your practice's overall capital. That is why so many dentists fail to see the merits of investing in the growth and development of their staff.

It is a fact that people look for opportunities to grow in their careers. No opportunity means that they will not stick around for very long.[32] When you lose a good employee, you lose all the training, time, and effort you have invested in them.

According to the Bureau of Labor Statistics,[33] people change jobs anywhere between 11 and 15 times in their lives.

---

32  Glenn Llopis, 10 Signs Your Employees Are Growing Complacent In Their Careers, http://www.forbes.com/sites/glennllopis/2013/07/08/10-signs-your-employees-are-growing-complacent-in-their-careers/

33  Alison, Doyle, How Often Do People Change Jobs?, http://jobsearch.about.com/od/employmentinformation/f/change-jobs.htm

Millennials are even worse—job hopping the moment they are unsatisfied. You need a plan of action to retain your employee investment.

Managing your human investment correctly means allowing room for continuous growth and development. An intern at your practice should be able to work their way up to office manager—if that is what they want.

Ongoing training might be an additional cost, but the long-term returns are justified. Imagine how much stronger that office manager would be if they worked their way up to that point from the intern level? These are the people you want to retain and nurture.

There are literally dozens of benefits that dentists rarely think about when the topic of ongoing staff training comes around.

It is your job to help your staff be as successful as they want to be, even though they work within your practice for a set salary.

- Room for growth is one of the single biggest motivators when starting a new job. Promotions and increased salaries always inspire higher quality work.

- Ongoing training ensures that each and every employee in your practice is 100% up to date on all the latest information, practices, and options available to your patients—which makes them a walking knowledge resource and customer service tool.

- Ongoing training can involve the development of certain skills[34] for overall performance improvement or expanding skills in areas like team work, customer service, and other extremely important areas.

- Your employees will contribute in a more pro-active

---

34  How Do I Contribute To An Employees Career Development, http://www.fsa.usda.gov/FSA/hrdapp?area=home&subject=mgrs&topic=ccd

manner to the growth and development of your practice when they are directly tied to it.

- The benefits trickle over into customer service, individual performance, and team dynamics—but most of all, to the continued expansion of your practice! A great office manager can break off and become a partner in your second practice for example.

These benefits are just some of the ways that the people in your practice will help you become the highly successful practice owner that you want to be.

A large part of the hiring process involves recruiting people that want to learn on a continuous basis, which means better career prospects for them down the line.

In order to keep your staff working towards the good of your practice, here are some great ways you can institute ongoing training.

- On-the-job training or orientation is a system that you will institute once a new employee joins your team. Another member of your staff and the office manager will train your new employee until they are comfortable with company practices.
- Offer your employees the opportunity to take courses through your practice to strengthen their current knowledge in certain areas. Short or long, these courses will attract your most ambitious employees. You can also make them compulsory.
- Seminars are often located in different areas, so it is an opportunity to take a few employees somewhere different for team building and knowledge growth. Try to attend as many local seminars as you can.

- Workshops and conferences are handy teaching tools, and there are many to choose from in their field of dentistry. Attend these in groups, and make sure that your employees soak up the knowledge and enjoy themselves.

- Create a side program for employees who want to become leaders[35] within your practice. Leadership education is now widespread, and you can do it online or at a local education center.

Stay on the lookout for new education opportunities for yourself and your employees. They will appreciate it, and more, it will bring you closer together. You cannot expect to have loyal patients if you cannot even create loyal employees!

---

35  How Well Do You Develop Your People?, http://www.mindtools.com/pages/article/team-development.htm

## chapter 12

# Supercharge Your Employees' Attitudes With Incentives

"Call it what you will, incentives are what get people to work harder."

NIKITA KHRUSHCHEV

Since the beginning of the drive to use big data to support organizational growth and development, there has been a shift to loyalty programs and staff incentive programs—because they have been proven to work.

Motivation in your everyday dental practice is the one thing that is often missing. Employees look tired, dentists look stressed and hurried, and no one seems like they really want to be there. That is why patients often never return.

It is also why you need to supercharge your employee attitudes with a nice incentive program. An incentive program or plan[36] can be defined as a performance plan that prompts exceptional behavior for a specific period of time, usually to achieve an objective.

---

36  Jerry Anderson, What Are Incentive Plans?, http://smallbusiness.chron.com/incentive-plans-1776.html

When you introduce incentives to your team, it inspires friendly competition and better team work and often helps you attain those key goals much quicker than you plan to.

That is why not having any incentive program right now is harming your practice. It is a trend that is sweeping through the medical niche, so your competitors are almost certainly using it—and the best employees are flocking to them.

Incentives can range from bonus cash incentives to small tokens, time off work, gifts, vacations, and anything worth working for. They are always above and beyond the scope of the employees' original salary requirements.

The question then becomes, should your dental practice create an incentive program for your employees? I would say yes, almost definitely.

Here are some solid reasons why your dental practice will benefit from your employees being incentivized a lot of the time:

- Sharing wealth, health, and happiness is always a good business practice, and when you are open to incentives for your employees, they see that you are interested in making their lives better too.

- Motivation nearly always wanes at certain times during the week. To keep these times strong, incentivize them and watch the difference!

- Incentive programs rapidly improve practice loyalty. When you award someone a four-day cruise vacation because they deserve it, they pay back the compliment.

- You get the benefit of having highly motivated employees working for you all the time, which means better patient service and better performance levels.

- Studies indicate that properly built incentive programs can increase employee performance by as much as 44%.[37]
- Employees are more willing to go beyond their job description when they know that you will be rewarding them for it.

There are many pitfalls involved in creating quality incentive programs—they can backfire and cause poor work performance, disagreements, and issues if you are not careful. It is best to keep your incentives program simple.

The latest research by the Total Rewards Association[38] indicates that 42% of all employees in their study agreed that incentives had a positive effect on employee engagement.

With patients, you, and your employees benefitting from incentives, it is clear that you need to seriously consider instituting a program in your practice. Here is how:

- Draft a simple incentives plan, and involve your employees. They must fully understand what the rules and regulations are for your rewards.
- All goals must be realistic and attainable, and they should be increased as they are achieved. If goals are reached quickly—or not at all—the incentive plan must be adjusted as needed.
- There should be incentives at all levels of your practice— for general employees and your management team.

37  The Incentives Research Foundation Resource Center, http://theirf.org/research/content/6000065/incentives-motivation-and-workplace-performance-research-and-best-practices/

38  Dr. Dow Scott, The Impact of Rewards Programs on Employee Engagement, http://www.worldatwork.org/waw/adimLink?id=39032

- Short-term and long-term incentives[39] are different, but they drive organizational growth if used correctly and concurrently.

- As a rule, no new employee is eligible for an incentive until they have been at your practice for longer than six months.

- You need to ensure that presentation of these incentives is done in honor of the individual receiving them; public congratulations do wonders for morale.

- One large reward at the end of the year can go to the employee that had the best work performance or data-based feedback at the end.

Make sure that your employees remain excited about their incentives by structuring them into small, medium, and large rewards. Small rewards will keep them going, and large rewards will keep them growing.

---

39  Team Incentive Bonus Plans, http://www.dentaleconomics.com/articles/print/volume-98/issue-5/features/team-incentive-bonus-plans.html

## chapter 13

# Communication Station: All Aboard

"The single biggest problem in communication is the illusion that it has taken place."

GEORGE BERNARD SHAW

Clear communication is easily the most vital reason why your practice is able to perform as it does. If it does not perform, chances are it is because of "unclear" communication.

At all levels, you need to ensure that communication with your dental patients is crystal clear so that you can act on what they really want from you.

No communicating is a common element found in dental practices. Pushy dentists try hard to sell treatments, and timid patients have terrible experiences.

There are many, many methods of improving doctor–patient communication in your practice. It all comes down to building communication systems founded on experiences that you know (and dentists that own thriving practices know) have worked in the past.

It is hard for the patient to communicate private details to you as an authority figure. That is why you need to make it obvious and easy for them to do so—by being warm, listening to their reservations, and addressing them.

Once you have boarded the train at communication station, word will get out that you are a modern dentist who wants to help. It all begins with honest, transparent communication.

Too many dentists pretend to communicate[40] with their patients but do not know the first thing about them. Unclear, rushed, or missed information can at best prompt a refund and at worst cause a lawsuit, so this is not something to take lightly.

Communication—even if you believe that yours is excellent—can always be improved. It takes more than just you to verify that your communication is good.

That is why you should be open to the idea that improved communication with your patients is something that must be integrated into your dental practice culture. Here is why.

- Clear communication reduces your margin of error and therefore reduces your overall risk profile when dealing with a patient. You understand them, they understand you, and no issues result.

- Practicing empathy is an excellent way to improve patient–doctor relationships and inspire trust in your practice and treatment options.

- Non-verbal communication like gestures and posture make all the difference to patient perception. Closing the door and giving them your full attention inspires loyalty, while chatting to other technicians, being on your phone, and reviewing patient records on your computer does not.

---

40  DDU, Dental Defense Union, http://www.theddu.com/press-centre/press-releases/ddu-advises-dental-professionals-to-communicate-clearly-with-patients

- Active listening involves hearing and understanding what your patient wants, not just preparing your counter-argument. Dentists that do this have lifetime patients.

- Pain measurement using verbal questions or structures helps the patient let you know how much they hurt—a very important thing to know.

- Follow up communication[41] and written communication is also important. Since when did dentists become too good to email their patients?

A lack of communication in any of these areas would result in a patient experiencing pain and discomfort and feeling like they are not important and not heard. Most of the time your patient will leave and never return.

There are multiple levels of communication to consider, and you are not a master of them all. Neither is your staff. That is why you need to institute a method of improving your communication with your patients.

- Focus on building a rapport with your patients—speak about work, school, community, their interests, their kids, and their area.

- Learn to listen effectively so that you can persuade your patient, provide diagnostic accuracy, and ensure a greater level of patient satisfaction.

- Listening involves giving your patient your full attention. Turn away from your computer, close the door, and put your chart down. It is patient communication time.

- Speak in an assertive and authoritative manner to your patient. Be humble, yet believe in the treatments you propose. Always have data to back up why it is needed.

---

41 Anyone Can Learn To Communicate Better, https://www.protectorplan.com/wp-content/uploads/documents/benefits/risk-management/Communication.pdf

- Practice explaining dental conditions,[42] and inform the patient what is going to happen and why. Involve them in the diagnostic process, and show them images and camera stills.

- Practice gently explaining the consequences of not following through with a procedure in a non-threatening manner.

- Focus on convincing patients to accept your treatment in a mutually beneficial way. Be real with your patient and frank about the process, the cost, and the outcomes.

Make patient communication a central part of your practice culture, and you will see how quickly people respond to the level of care that they deserve.

---

42  Top 10 Skills For Success In Dental Communication, http://www.ncdental. org/images/ncds/Wright%20-%20Top%2010%20Skills%20for%20Success%20 in%20Dental%20Communication.pdf

# More Than Just Lip Service
## *(Customer Relationship Strategy)*

## chapter 14

# The Right Customer Is Always Right

"The aim of marketing is to know and understand the customer so well the product or service fits him and sells itself."

PETER DRUCKER

As a dentist, it is your job to fix teeth, sure, but it is also your job to sell cosmetic treatments like veneers, teeth whitening, and gap filling.

In order to do this effectively, you need to institute a customer relationship strategy, or as I like to call it, a "patient relationship strategy" to keep your practice lucrative.

I honestly do not understand why there is such secrecy about cosmetic treatments in dentistry. All that leads to is unhappy patients and bad reputations for dentists.

Instead, why not target your ideal patient and learn how to convert them over and over again. It makes sense in other businesses, so why not your practice? The fact is that thriving practices understand their value to the patient as well as the lifetime value of the patient to their practice.

If you think your patient will only ever want restorative work, you may never have a thriving practice. One of my thriving dentists spends a good deal of time just getting to know the patient. Where do they shop? What kind of car do they drive? Where do they live? Where do their kids go to school? This tells a lot more about the personality of the patient than "Where does it hurt?" Next, this thriving dentist hands the patient a large mirror and asks the patient to look closely in the mirror and then tell him everything they see that they do not like.

Much of that information will not be dealt with for some time. But if there is a little composite that can be put on a canine to restore a little balance as well as temporarily improve function and wear then he will do it right then. He also looks for low cost value added services that he can do for free to help establish trust and rapport as well as build some good will with a new patient.

This might be giving the patient EXTRA samples of oral rinse products or a new bleaching tray. The concept of reciprocity is alive and well with this practice.

A large part of keeping your patients happy is making them feel special. This means getting them to become a long-term patient of yours and ticking all the boxes when it comes to prevention, treatment, and cosmetic options.

When you treat a single patient as a consistent revenue stream, guess what? It improves levels of transparency, honesty, and trust in your practice. Then that patient will go out into the world and, via word of mouth,[43] get you more patients.

No more sucking up or demanding treatments from patients out of need. No more low conversion direct selling. There are lots of other ways to have a successful doctor–patient relationship in dentistry.

---

43  Kristie Nation, Social Media – It's Just Word of Mouth Marketing!, http://www.dentaleconomics.com/articles/print/volume-103/issue-2/technology-needs/social-media-its-just-word-of-mouth-marketing.html

The right customer will pay you on time, will always choose elective procedures, and will be thrilled with your work and your practice.

These are the individuals that you want telling other people about your practice. That means keeping them happy, but it also means understanding if they are not.

Here are some great reasons why the right patient is always a good investment but the wrong patient will detract from what you are trying to build:

- It is a myth that dentists cannot choose their patients. Sometimes it will not feel right, in which case you can refer them to another dentist who will suit them better. When you do this, you make way for patients who love your work.
- The right patients have a higher chance of being happy with your work and therefore will not cost you money or waste your time.
- The right patient personas[44] will always recommend your practice to other patients when they are looking for someone like you.
- The right patients brighten up your day, give you that sense of community contribution, and help you be the best at your job.
- The right patient can afford your services, is happy to pay your prices, and will be eager to undergo any elective treatments that improve their dental health.

While it is not common to turn patients away when they are in need, they are not the focus of your practice community

44  Rob Lovitt, Look Who's Talking: Patient Personas Can Provide Invaluable Insights, http://medibeauty.biz/look-whos-talking-patient-personas-can-provide-invaluable-insights/

either. When you shift your attention to the clients that really matter, you can improve revenue, attendance, scheduled cleans, and more.

## SANDRA GREGG

Senior Sales, Management and Marketing Consultant at PractiDent Worldwide, believes:

*"Delivering superior customer service that exceeds patient expectations will ensure enhanced treatment acceptance and patient referrals. In most dental marketplaces today, there is competition for attracting and retaining patients, and it is critical to remember that in most cases, exceptional customer service is truly the only thing that differentiates you from your competitors."*

Keeping the right dental patients happy will result in a boost for your practice. That is why I encourage you to focus on long-term patients in your practice.

Comfort is a huge patient concern. Make sure that your waiting rooms are comfortable, relaxing, and pleasant.

Institute a patient rewards program that provides discounts to repeat patients. It will inspire loyalty and repeat business in your practice.

Learn to address the core concerns with treatment planning—time, money, and fear. Create easy-to-consume media around these areas for your patient personas.

Make your patient feel special by getting them to sign up to your online email list or app. Send them personalized messages on special occasions and discount gifts.

Get your ideal patients involved in a referral program. For every patient they refer, give them a nice discount or a reward. It works, and they love it.

Educate to motivate[45] your patients by investing heavily in online content, education media, and other tools for keeping your patients thinking about you.

Use various dental practice touch points to collect data, then analyze the feedback to see where your service profile needs work.

Keep your dental office clean, odor free, and modern to create a positive climate for your patients. If your practice looks good, you are friendly and efficient, AND you have a patient rewards program, you can turn any patient into a long-term source of income.

---

45  10 Proven Steps To Receive More Patients, http://dentalpracticesolutions.com/blog/2010/02/01/10-proven-steps-to-receive-more-patients/

## chapter 15

# Great Expectations and How to Manage Them

"If you paint in your mind a picture of bright and happy expectations, you put yourself into a condition conducive to your goal."

NORMAN VINCENT PEALE

A crucial part of guaranteeing good patient relations involves the ability to set, manage, and monitor patient expectations.

A patient will march into your offices and will have a list of needs that have to be fulfilled. It is your job to be able to fulfill them and to exceed the patient's expectations.

There is a fresh opportunity to do this every time a new patient enters your offices. Expectations are a funny thing. Some patients only expect to leave pain free. Others expect full service treatment and lavender towels after their filling is done.

Expectations become a key concern when treatment options[46] for your patient are involved. This is also why communication

---

46 Managing Patient Expectations, http://www.dental-risk.com/Portals/20/ articles/Patient%20Expectations.pdf

is so important. You need to be able to talk them through every process to ensure that what they expect is in line with reality.

I have heard stories of outraged mothers calling dentists to demand their money back because their child's tooth is still sore after a root canal. This is not the child's fault; it is the dentist's fault for not letting the mother know that tenderness is a part of the healing process.

---

**ALLAN G. FARMAN**

Professor of Radiology and Imaging Science at University of Louisville Health Sciences Center, says,

*"Treatment failure is to be expected occasionally as we are all human. Key to minimizing failure is to use methods that you are pretty certain will work rather than just hope may work. Key to minimizing unwanted events following failure are (1) to discuss possible failures with the patient in advance rather than giving false expectations and (2) taking care of failures when they do occur rather than pretending they did not happen."*

---

With great expectations comes great responsibility—and as the dentist, they rest squarely on your shoulders. Treatment processes must be patient-centric for this reason.

In both restorative and cosmetic work, you will need to have systems of communication in place that deal with patient expectations.

There are many good reasons to focus on reliable and responsible methods of managing patient expectations in your practice. If expectations are not met, you will almost certainly lose that patient. There are a number of factors to consider with cosmetic and repair services:

- Dentists can be criticized and complaints can be made against them because expectations were not met. This is not to be confused with poor service delivery.

- Patients might refuse to pay for treatments, which will lose you money, or they may decide to broadcast what a "rip off" you are to the entire Internet.

- Sometimes patients will demand that you redo the work, which means that you have to spend your time and money repeating a standard service outcome because you failed to inform the patient.

- With elective cosmetic treatments[47] this is even more important. They are often expensive, which means that if patients do not get what they are expecting—or if they suffer any side effects—you will get into trouble.

- A smile, for example is a highly personal thing to work on; you can set appropriate expectations for it using technology.

- The general rule with dentistry, as with any business, is to under promise and over deliver because this model always guarantees satisfaction from your patient.

With these reasons, you cannot ignore the eternal need for adequate expectation management—from you and your dental staff.

How do you go about ensuring that your patient expectations are met every single time? Well, you have already done a lot by systematizing your processes.

What remains is to ensure that your people, planning, and preparation are also taken care of, as they are part of the expectation management cycle.

---

47  Marc Montgomery, Predictably Meeting Patient's Expectations In Esthetic Dentistry, http://www.oralhealthgroup.com/news/predictably-meeting-patients-expectations-in-esthetic-dentistry/1001044208/?&er=NA

- Financial expectations can be sorted out using the right software and by being verbally transparent with your patient before every procedure.

- Guarantees and warranties must be discussed before you do any sort of work for a new patient. For some reason, patients expect you to guarantee your work, but you are not a mechanic or a baker.

- Make sure that before your staff get your patients to sign anything, a discussion about expectations[48] is held. This must be part of your policy.

- Use modern technology like video simulation software to show patients what they can expect to look like after a cosmetic procedure. This will help them make the right choices and will help reduce dissatisfaction.

- Use your various online media to educate your patients about your policies and procedures. Structure your website as a learning resource that is specific to your patient list.

With the right strategy, employee commitment, and preparation on your end, every single patient will fully understand every process, service, or outcome that you provide. That is all your patients can expect from you.

---

48  Michael Young, Managing Patient Expectations, http://www.prodentalcpd.com/UserFiles/File/Articles/Business/P513_managing_patient_expectations.pdf

## chapter 16

# Online Education Media for Patient Retention

"Going online and asking questions is
the best way to learn."

TOM FELTON

Your dental patients come from all sorts of backgrounds and circumstances. When they are not at your practice, they are out there in the world, living their lives.

So how do you reach them when they are not in need of dental treatment? The answer is simple: online education media.

It is a harsh fact now that dental practices that are not on the Internet do not get as many patients. People expect you to be there—and more, they expect you to be creating all sorts of content for their benefit.

Small business owners call it "value-added" content, or content that serves to educate and inspire your dental patients to use you again.

It is a type of inbound marketing[49] that will attract new and existing patients to you without any direct face-to-face contact at all.

This is mostly done using your online web presence—a key element in your current dental practice's marketing arsenal.

If you want to retain patients and convert them into lifelong, repeat business, you cannot overlook the benefits of investing money into your online brand identity.

---

**TORREY GAGE**

Executive Vice President at Think Big Go Local, says:

*"We have been using the combination of reputation marketing, social media marketing, video marketing, and more to achieve 'celebrity' status for our clients since our inception. For a dentist, steps that could be taken to become an authority could include participating in HARO (Help a Reporter), hosting a podcast or Google Hangouts show, becoming a contributing expert at AllExperts.com, having a book on dentistry ghost written and published on Kindle, or having 'interview style' videos made, etc."*

---

Service businesses like yours need constant booking, and that means you need constant interaction and engagement with your patients.

To be left behind with modern marketing practices like social media and content marketing will do nothing for your practice. The bottom line is that your competitors are using it, and they are taking your patients from you.

---

49  Health Services Success Story: Legacy Dental, http://www.hubspot.com/customers/legacy-dental

Here are some reasons why you should focus on your online presence:

- Having a community around your brand online not only increases patient education, it builds a reputation shield around you for those times when people speak out against your brand.
- Providing consistent education resources to your patients online is a way to secure your authority and credibility in your niche.
- Creating content resources like videos, podcasts, and blog posts is a great way to promote long-term patient loyalty—which compounds when you add customer relationship and loyalty programs to that list.
- When you secure the best online presence and when people search for dentists[50] in your area, you will come up. Then it is up to your identity to get them into your offices.
- Creating content for your niche not only positions you as an expert, it positions every staff member inside your practice as part of a solid expert team. That is powerful!

With a dedicated social media manager, you have an in-house content creator that will help you maintain these online properties, strategies, and needs.

Knowing how to go about setting up your online presence is as important as deciding to have one. That is why I have mapped out a simple process that will work for you.

- Approach a digital strategy company, and enlist the help of someone to establish your online brand strategy.

---

50   Shauna Duty, How To Win Traffic and Influence Rankings, http://moderndentalmarketing.com/category/content-marketing-2/

- Get a website created for your dental practice with community-centric features like a blog and a forum area. Live chat is also being used increasingly.

- Get your social media manager (you need to hire one) to create a social strategy for you centered around your blog. Identify which social properties you need to be on, and then establish yourself there.

- Create a content strategy to populate your websites and social properties on an ongoing basis. Unique content like videos, blog posts, infographics, and podcasts get shared the most—and you want your content to be shared!

- Using social media marketing, content marketing,[51] and real time engagement, you can generate passive income on your websites while pulling in new patients and converting more old patients with your education resources.

- Additional Internet marketing features likes apps, SMS, and games should be explored with a digital strategist.

If you take the time to build a quality online presence and system for reaching out to patients on the Internet, you will not have to do any real world marketing. That will save you time and money and will take a whole lot of pressure off your staff.

---

51 Al Lautenslager, Content Marketing For Doctors, Dentists and Practices, http://www.slideshare.net/algtr17/content-marketing-for-doctors-dentists-and-practices

chapter 17

# Creating a Climate of Trust: Fairness and Transparency in Practice

"A lie can travel half way around the world while the truth is putting on its shoes."

CHARLES SPURGEON

Perhaps the most overlooked element in patient relationship management is concerned with trust building. If there is no trust that exists between doctor and patient, then you cannot expect loyalty, respect, or anything more than fly-by-night patients.

A key part of this is communication, but we have dealt with that. When you define what trust actually means to the average patient, it clarifies a lot.

Trust builds solid foundations for long-term patient care. From the patient's perspective, they want a dentist who is priced fairly, highly competent, compassionate, gentle, and willing to do extra work in order to keep the patient pain-free, comfortable, and solvent.

Of course, trust is built around putting the patient first. That is a hard thing to do when competitors are around and bills need to be paid.

But let me be clear about it—if you do not factor trust into your practice business strategy, then it will not be of primary concern. And it should be!

Trust is also about checking all the boxes—with honesty, transparency, finances, and personal wellbeing. If you trust your patient to be upfront with you, you owe them the same.

Three prominent methods of guaranteeing trust fall under ethics,[52] communication, and shared decision-making. Again, you have to put the needs of your patient first.

Did you know that some 80%[53] of all U.S. adults have some form of dental anxiety? It does not end there. Patients see dentist rooms as hostile places. They are afraid to make appointments and even more nervous about speaking to their dentists.

This is why it is so essential that you focus on building trust with your patients. Here are some great reasons to do so:

- Trust cannot exist in a climate of fear, and dental anxiety is a real fear. A big part of your job is making sure that your patient's fears are addressed and alleviated.

- Trust is even more important when your patient is in pain and in a vulnerable position. You must put systems in place to uphold this trust.

- Trust has been in question in the dental industry as medical aids have changed and patients are not sure about what they can and cannot afford. Helping them through this process will build instant trust.

- If a patient trusts you, they are more likely to recommend you online or tell their friends and family about you in person.

---

52  Jeremy Jacquot, Trust In The Dentist-Patient Relationship: A Review, http://www.jyi.org/issue/trust-in-the-dentist-patient-relationship-a-review/

53  Michael Liu, The Dentist/Patient Relationship: The Role of Dental Anxiety, http://scholarship.claremont.edu/cgi/viewcontent.cgi?article=1253&context=cmc_theses

- When your patient trusts your practice, they will make you their first choice every single time they have to endure a dental procedure.

Good experiences are really the only thing that a patient cares about with regard to trust. They can forgive nearly anything but treatment quality and care. Make sure that you look after your patients and are a supportive, reliable dentist.

Trust is built on ethical behavior and intentions. If you can build trust practices into your business, you will benefit in the long term, and your patient retention rates will skyrocket.

Here is how you can focus on building trust in your practice:

- Make sure that your office employees keep all patient information private and confidential to put their minds at ease.

- Directly address a nervous patient and alleviate their mistrust verbally by walking them through the process. If they appear too afraid, stop. Orientate yourself, discuss it, and then move forward again.

- Always make sure that your patient cannot feel pain before you begin the procedure. No pain wins half the battle already, so do not assume a quiet patient is pain free.

- Always deliver what you promise, and never make promises that you cannot keep. Stick to vague descriptions when working with cosmetics and tell the patient that you will do your best but all treatments result in slight variations.

- Clean, friendly employees that treat your patients with respect will always be trusted, but most of the trust will come from your end.

- Be frank about costs, honest about procedures,[54] and really help your patient weigh up if they need certain treatments. Be a guide, not a salesman.

Most of all, trust takes time. That is why you need an online presence—so that your patients can grow to trust you more, even when they are not around.

54  Rosemary Rowe, Michael Calnan, Trust Relations in Healthcare – The New Agenda, http://eurpub.oxfordjournals.org/content/16/1/4.full

## chapter 18

# Flexibility and the Art of Structured Payments

*"The boldness of asking deep questions may require unforeseen flexibility if we are to accept the answers."*

BRIAN GREENE

We live in the Internet age, which means that not only do people expect a certain level of flexibility now, but they are fully aware of their other options—often to your detriment.

That is why it has become more important than ever to make sure that you run through all treatments options with your patients: ones that you do and ones that you do not do.

Chances are, some patients will know about the other options, and they may assume that your omission means that you are after their money, not their best interests.

That said, patients also expect a certain level of flexibility with payment concerns these days, especially in light of the recent insurance changes in the U.S.

Why is it that you can walk into any clothing store and get a thousand dollars credit, but when you really need it, you cannot do the same at your local dentist?

Times are changing, and your method of structuring payments also needs to change. Flexibility is becoming a modern differentiator, one that meets the needs of patients that have nowhere else to turn but will gladly pay interest for the service.

First, you should be upfront about all the different treatment options there are. Then you need to be transparent about your different payment structures. If you handle this right, you can accommodate your patients in times of great need, and this is not quickly forgotten in a community.

There are many reasons why you need to consider being more flexible with your treatment and payment options in this economic climate. Here are a few:

- Your patients can choose from 20 other dentists in your area if they feel that you are not giving them the flexibility in service[55] or payment that they require.

- For every payment that you refuse, there is a modern dentist around the corner who is profiting off your stubborn inability to accept different payment structures.

- Sometimes a patient will need to think about a treatment before having it. If they go home and find out other options are available—and better options—they will lose faith in you and never return.

- When you give your patient a full list of thorough options, they see it as a customer service, one that reinforces the patient–doctor bond and inspires repeat business.

- Finances are a sticky subject for many patients. When you approach them about it, it is far more comfortable than leaving it to them to ask. Many patients would rather

---

55  The List: Top 7 Products Patients Demand, http://www.dentalproductsreport. com/dental/article/list-top-7-products-patients-demand

refuse the treatment than leave to look for cheaper options elsewhere.

Flexibility is not something that dentists are widely known for; in fact, it is a rarity in the medical industry. This makes it a key differentiation for your practice—one that could end up being the reason why your patient list is always full and happy.

So how do you go about ensuring that your dental practice lives up to patient demand for multiple service options and multiple payment structures?

- Conduct research on the service profiles of the dentists in your area to make sure that you offer those "extra" services patients cannot get elsewhere.

- Always be willing to help your patient find the treatment they need if you do not offer it. They will return to you again if you do.

- Investigate various payment options and plans for your patient. Consider Visa, MasterCard, and EFT payments.

- Take a closer look at discounted cash payments or payment plans that patients can sign for when they are at your offices.

- Split payment structures, in-house financing, and accepting online payments are a few more ideas to get you moving forward.

- Chat with your financial advisor and accountant about the various payment options[56] you can afford to offer, and structure them so that you never have to deal with cash shortfall.

---

56 Paying For Dental Care, http://www.mouthhealthy.org/en/dental-care-concerns/paying-for-dental-care/

Speak to your patients about the various options and payment flexibility that they need. Let them know that your practice is all about customized dental solutions for the people in your community. That is how you win the hearts, minds, and wallets of your patients!

If you are unsure about the payment structures, test them using your in-house CRM software. If after a few months they are not working, change them.

# Leveraging Unique Opportunities With Each Patient

"Opportunity is missed by most people because it is dressed in overalls and looks like work."

THOMAS A. EDISON

Each of your patients will be different and have a unique set of problems—which presents a unique set of opportunities when you see them. Knowing how to leverage these unique opportunities will help you generate income and keep your patients happy.

Some dental patients will have a very simple set of needs—a cleaning and the odd filling. Others will have multiple issues, root canals, and damage to fix. Still others will only be in your offices to seek out cosmetic fixes.

Each of these patients presents new opportunities for you as a dentist who is looking to gain long-term, repeat business. You should have an evaluation system[57] in place for new patients

---

57  Patient Assessment, http://www.dentalcare.com/en-US/dental-education/ continuing-education/ce393/ce393.aspx?ModuleName=coursecontent&PartID=1 &SectionID=-1

and an assessment process for existing patients, based on their past histories.

The opportunities I am talking about relate to conversion and patient happiness. You should have a long-term treatment plan ready to propose to these individual patient personas.

When you get to know your dental practice well enough, it becomes clear how your patient lists should be segmented. You can use these to predefine services to sell to your patients.

Opportunities are not unethical methods of converting patients into money; they are ways for you to provide a higher level of service to your patient while still meeting their needs. That is why you need to consider these reasons for leveraging patient opportunities:

- Some patients may have special healthcare[58] needs and would benefit from a much more supportive environment for their own safety. Recommending this is not only ethical but you can refer the patient to a network partner.

- Assess patient risk in order to provide them with the best possible treatment options. Then care pathways can be defined, and together you can build a treatment plan that works for both of you.

- Preventing things like gum disease and other dental issues is important in patient planning. Come up with a custom prevention plan for your patient, and make sure that they stick to it for their own benefit.

- Collecting various forms of feedback from your patients will give you the data you need to streamline your offerings.

Opportunities in the form of treatments, preventative measures, referrals, product sales, and more can present

---

58  Guidelines on Management of Dental Patients With Special Health Care Needs, http://www.aapd.org/media/Policies_Guidelines/G_SHCN.pdf

themselves on a day-to-day basis. When a hairdresser recommends shampoo, no one minds, and it is the same with you. I have always found it ironic that toothpastes say "recommended by dentists," but there are still dental practices that do not sell preventative products to patients.

How do you leverage unique opportunities? By being able to identify them! All you need to do is come up with scenarios where different treatment, referral, or product offerings would be relevant and helpful.

- Create assessment criteria for patients that need to focus more on preventing their next cavity or reducing the chance of getting a serious disease.
- If a patient meets the criteria, offer them a treatment package or a product based on the fact that it will help them avoid future dentist visits.
- Learn to leverage technology to support these efforts. An example may be product displays on your monitors in-house or sending text reminders to your patients to floss twice a week!
- Use real world patient testimonials on your websites and social channels[59] to show the world that you put your patients first.
- Network with other dentists and medical professionals and see if you can work out a method of referral that benefits your practice.
- Always give honest, professional advice to your patients, and never exploit them. Sales are only all right when it is in line with your patient's needs.

---

59  Roger Levin, Leverage Your Most Powerful Source For New Dental Patients, http://www.dentistryiq.com/articles/2013/02/leverage-your-most-powerful-source-for-new-dental-patients.html

Make a point of continually looking out for opportunities to recommend products or services, or—indeed—treatment options that will benefit your patients and support your bottom line.

## chapter 20

# Being the Heart of Your Patient–Practitioner Relationship

"Customer satisfaction is worthless.
Customer loyalty is priceless."

JEFFREY GITOMER

There are lots of factors that go into being a world class dentist. Not every kid that makes it through dental school is going to be a successful dentist.

Researchers at Case Western Reserve University School of Dental Medicine[60] have conducted studies that indicate emotional intelligence could be to blame. It is more important in the doctor–patient relationship than previously thought.

Knowing how to manage your emotions and the emotions of your patient is critical in establishing long-term, mutually beneficial relationships. You have to be the heart of your relationship because you are the authority figure guiding them through their torrid dental journey.

---

60  Karen Fox, Emotional Intelligence Trumps IQ in Dentist-Patient Relationship, https://www.ada.org/news/8623.aspx

The dentists that do this best make a lot of money. The ones that do not tend to lose patients in droves. You need to become the kind of dentist that truly cares.

There are many factors to consider in this process, but you need to get your head around the fact that compassion, care, and emotional connection are needed in your career.

For too long the image of the heartless dentist has damaged your self-perception. Before treatment, before medicine, comes your very real relationship with your long-term patients. If you can get this right, you stand to become one of the most successful practices in your city, perhaps even in your state, if you follow a growth model.

The average dentist has a network of contacts in hospitals, among specialists, and with technologists all over their area. But what about their patients?

Here are some reasons to create a relationship building program:

- Your patients will judge you on who you are, how you treat them, and what you are prepared to do to accommodate them. This has nothing to do with how good you are at your treatments and practices.

- The better you are at connecting with your patients, the more likely they are to heed your advice and listen to your treatment plan. This helps when you are trying to sell them a product or treatment that will solve their problem.

- Trust is formed when a patient feels real emotional connection[61] from you, which means that they are more likely to recommend you to others and return to use you if they ever have another dental concern.

61  Iris Tse, In Better Health: Doctor-Patient Relationships Show Improvement, http://www.livescience.com/13014-doctor-patient-relationships-improving.html

- Being a compassionate dentist is about caring how your patient feels before, during, and after treatment. Support them as best you can, and they will feel no pain and no emotional distress, and they will have a pleasant, comfortable experience.

If you can work on your patient relationships to the point where you personally know the bulk of your patients, it will only work in your favor. There is no such thing as impersonal dentistry anymore. You can try to succeed, but it will not work very well.

You will need to take steps personally and in your practice to become the kind of dentist who puts your patients first. Connection and true relationships need to be nurtured often, even if it is from afar.

Here is how you should practice improving your doctor–patient relationship:

- Think about instituting a peer review program[62] at your practice, where your performance with patients is assessed. This will help you improve in the long term.

- Institute a patient loyalty program that provides unique benefits to your patients based on their needs, like product discounts for example.

- Spend time getting to know each patient, and make a point of revisiting their file before they arrive so that you can refresh on who they are.

- Practice empathetic responses to your patient and appropriate levels of concern when they talk directly to you.

- When patients have questions, go to great lengths to make them understand what the answers are.

---

62 Dentistry's Dispute Resolution Program, http://www.ada.org/sections/professionalResources/pdfs/Peer_Review_Brochure.pdf

• Leverage online media to chat and improve relationships with your patients while blogging or on social media sites.

Begin looking for ways to improve your relationships, and soon it will become second nature to you. Write down any good ideas that you have, and try to make them practice policy.

If you know you have trouble with irritability and are not a "people person," I advise you to take some acting classes where they can help you with that. It sounds unconventional, but it is what the pros do when they need to rid themselves of social anxiety!

# Conclusion

With these 20 powerful dental practices, you will transform your business into what you always knew that it could be.

Dentists these days need to be aware that their patients no longer have to visit them on a regular basis. Shopping around happens a lot, and few people have time anymore for cold, mechanical dentists that do not care.

Your competitors have realized this and so have larger dental institutions. Steps must be taken to ensure the solvency and survival of your practice. My hope is that this book has given you a wealth of information to process and that you cannot wait to write all of your ideas down.

Remember, you have two doors to your practice: the front door and the back door. Thriving practices lock the back door and widen the front door.

Transforming your practice requires a brave heart. You must realize that there are no sacred cows. Either everyone is on board or you need to throw them overboard. Your thriving practice is right in front of you.

All it takes is a focus on the four core strategies that I have mentioned here: your personal self-development strategy, your treatment strategy, employee strategy, and customer relationship strategy. Get these right, and you cannot go wrong.

It takes people, process, patients, and personal investment to own and run a successful dental practice. You have the tools—now go thrive.

To your success,

*Michael Hill*

# References

**CHAPTER 1**

*Attitude Quotes*, BrainyQuote, http://www.brainyquote.com/quotes/topics/topic_attitude.html

Harrell, Keith, *Why Your Attitude is Everything*, http://www.success.com/article/why-your-attitude-is-everything

Cherry, Kendra, *How Attitudes Form, Change and Shape Our Behavior*, http://psychology.about.com/od/socialpsychology/a/attitudes.htm

Parnami, Kavya, *10 Reasons Why Having Positive Attitude and Outlook Towards Life Is Important*, http://listdose.com/10-reasons-positive-attitude-outlook-towards-life-important/

Myers, Teena, *The Importance of a Positive Attitude*, http://blog.nola.com/faith/2012/05/the_importance_of_a_positive_a.html

*Self-Affirmation Enhances Performance, Makes Us Receptive To Our Mistakes*, https://www.psychologicalscience.org/index.php/news/releases/self-affirmation-enhances-performance-makes-us-receptive-to-our-mistakes.html

**CHAPTER 2**

*Quotes on Vision*, http://www.leadershipnow.com/visionquotes.html

Ebben, Jay, *Developing Effective Mission and Vision Statements*, http://www.inc.com/resources/startup/articles/20050201/missionstatement.html

Collins, James, *Building Your Company's Vision*, http://hbr. org/1996/09/building-your-companys-vision/ar/1

Hom, Elaine, *What Is a Vision Statement*, http://www. businessnewsdaily.com/3882-vision-statement.html

Evans, Jennell, *Vision and Mission – What's The Difference and Why Does It Matter?*, http://www.psychologytoday.com/blog/ smartwork/201004/vision-and-mission-whats-the-difference-and-why-does-it-matter

*4 Reasons Why You Need a Personal Vision Statement*, http://www. collegefashion.net/college-life/personal-vision-statement/

**CHAPTER 3**

*Brand Quotes*, BrainyQuote, http://www.brainyquote.com/quotes/ keywords/brand.html

Reynolds, Siimon, *How You Can Build a Great Personal Brand*, http:// www.forbes.com/sites/siimonreynolds/2014/02/06/how-you-can-build-a-great-personal-brand/

Schawbel, Dan, *Personal Branding 101: How To Discover and Create Your Brand*, http://mashable.com/2009/02/05/personal-branding-101/

*What Is Personal Branding and Why Is It So Important?*, https://www. aspireforsuccess.com/what-branding-is.php

Montoya, Peter, *What Is Personal Branding?*, http://www. petermontoya.com/pdfs/tbcy-chapter1.pdf

Arruda, William, *7 Questions To Ask When Uncovering Your Personal Brand*, http://www.forbes.com/sites/williamarruda/2013/11/12/7-questions-to-ask-when-uncovering-your-personal-brand/

Hori, Roxanne, *The Importance of Managing Your Personal Brand*, http://www.businessweek.com/articles/2013-11-22/the-importance-of-managing-your-personal-brand

Chau, Lisa, *The Keys To Good Personal Branding*, http://www.usnews. com/opinion/blogs/economic-intelligence/2013/11/05/dore-clark-explains-the-importance-of-personal-branding

## CHAPTER 4

*Connection Quote*, BrainyQuote, http://www.brainyquote.com/quotes/keywords/connection.html

Levin, Roger, *Developing Lifetime Relationships With Patients: Strategies To Improve Patient Care and Build Your Practice*, http://www.dentalcare.com/media/en-US/research_db/pdf/jcdp/levinjan08.pdf

*Thursday Troubleshooter: Dental Patient Won't Complete Medical Forms*, http://www.dentistryiq.com/articles/2013/12/thursday-troubleshooter1.html

Joyal, Fred, *7 Real-Life Reasons Your Patients Leave*, http://www.1800dentist.com/7-reallife-reasons-your-patients-leave/

Sbaraini, Alexandra, Carter, Stacy, *Experiences of Dental Care: What Do Patient's Value*, http://www.biomedcentral.com/1472-6963/12/177

McMaster, Robert, *Practical Considerations For Treating The Anxious Dental Patient*, http://www.oralhealthgroup.com/news/practical-considerations-for-treating-the-anxious-dental-patient/1000880281/?&er=NA

Oeding, Mary, *Anxious or Phobic Patients: Best Treatment Practices*, http://www.dentallearning.org/course/Anxious_Phobic/Anxious%20Phobic%20Patients.pdf

## CHAPTER 5

*Pace Quotes*, BrainyQuotes, http://www.brainyquote.com/quotes/keywords/pace.html

*Preparation and Time Management*, http://www.ada.org/5439.aspx

*Time Management Tips For Dentists To Increase Work Efficiency*, http://schustercenter.com/practice-management/time-management-tips-for-dentists-to-increase-work-efficiency/

*How Health Coaching Can Improve Dental Care*, http://www.axiumdental.com/how-health-coaching-can-improve-dental-care/

*Dental Practice-Based Research To Improve Oral Health and To Support The Adoption of Evidence Based Clinical Practice*, http://www.nidcr.

nih.gov/GrantsAndFunding/See_Funding_Opportunities_Sorted_
By/ConceptClearance/CurrentCC/PracticeBasedResearch.htm

## CHAPTER 6

*Impression Quotes*, BrainyQuote, http://www.brainyquote.com/
quotes/keywords/impression.html

Knight, Renee, *Products For an Efficient Dental Practice and Enhanced
Patient Experience [Video]*, http://www.dentalproductsreport.com/
dental/article/products-efficient-dental-practice-and-enhanced-
patient-experience-video

*Knowing What Your Patients Want From You: The Importance of Making
Them Feel Special*, http://www.dentaleconomics.com/articles/print/
volume-100/issue-2/features/knowing-what-your-patients-want-
from-you-the-importance-of-making-them-feel-special.html

Joyal, Fred, *Five Steps To Making Your Dental Office Fun*, http://
www.1800dentist.com/five-steps-to-making-your-dental-office-fun/

*Survey: What Patients Like About Dental Office Experience*, http://
www.dentistryiq.com/articles/2012/12/survey-what-do-patients-
like-about-dental-offices.html

Henry, Kevin, *Convenience, Honesty, and Online Reviews…Some Of
The Things Your Dental Patients Want*, http://www.dentistryiq.com/
articles/2013/05/convenience--honesty--and-online-reviews-----
some-of-the-things-.html

## CHAPTER 7

*Consistency Quotes*, BrainyQuote, http://www.brainyquote.com/
quotes/keywords/consistency.html

*Creating Standards For Consistent, High Quality Dental Therapy
Education in The United States*, http://www.communitycatalyst.org/
doc-store/publications/dt-education-report-summary.pdf

*Quality Measurement in Dentistry: A Guidebook*, http://www.ada.org/
sections/dentalPracticeHub/pdfs/DQA_Guidebook_52913.pdf

Dykman, April, *Systematizing Your Startup 101*, http://mixergy.com/
systemizing-your-startup-101-resource-page/

*How To Systematize Your Business So Everything Will Run Smoothly, Even When You're Out of The Office,* http://mixergy.com/cheat-sheet-8-ways-to-systemize-your-business-so-everything-will-run-smoothly-even-when-you%E2%80%99re-out-of-the-office/

*How To Systematize Your Business: The First Step,* http://entrepreneursystems.com/2010/12/how-to-systemize-your-business-the-first-step/

## CHAPTER 8

*Quotes About Differentiation,* http://www.goodreads.com/quotes/tag/differentiation

*Differentiating On Customer Service? What Are The Key Issues?,* http://www.customerchampions.co.uk/differentiating-on-customer-service-what-are-the-key-issues/

Bashara, Timothy, *Three Ways To Differentiate Your Dental Practice From The Competition,* http://www.dentistryiq.com/articles/2013/11/three-ways-to-differentiate-your-practice-from-the-competition.html

Armstrong, James, Boardman, Anthony, *Eight Steps For Strategic Analysis Dental Practices,* http://www.cda-adc.ca/jcda/vol-65/issue-10/553.html

Pak, Jane, *Differentiated Dentists,* http://www.huffingtonpost.com/jane-pak/dentists-business_b_1546202.html

Deborah, H, *Differentiate Your Dental Practice From The Competition,* http://dentainment.com/differentiate-dental-practice/

Soloman, Eric, *The Future of Dentistry,* http://www.dentaleconomics.com/articles/print/volume-94/issue-11/features/the-future-of-dentistry.html

Nash, Kent, *Geographic Distribution of Dentists in The United States, American Dental Association, 2009 Distribution of Dentists in the U.S. by Region and State* http://www.ada.org/1444.aspx

## CHAPTER 9

*Leverage Quotes,* BrainyQuote, http://www.brainyquote.com/quotes/

keywords/leverage.html

*New Patient Loyalty Program Helps Dentists 'Beat Recession' Launches At ADA Annual Session,* http://www.loyalpatientsinc.com/pdf/Dental%20Product%20Reports%20October%2020%202008%20Launch%20of%20Patient%20Program.pdf

*Your Guide To Private Dentistry,* http://www.oft.gov.uk/shared_oft/consumer_leaflets/general/oft660.pdf

Beyers, Richard, *Evidence-Based Dentistry: A General Practitioner's Perspective,* https://www.cda-adc.ca/jcda/vol-65/issue-11/620.html

## CHAPTER 10

*Quotes About Hiring People,* http://www.chalre.com/hiring_managers/recruiting_quotes.htm

Rossheim, John, *How To Hire Office Staff For a Medical or Dental Practice,* http://hiring.monster.com/hr/hr-best-practices/recruiting-hiring-advice/acquiring-job-candidates/how-to-hire-office-staff.aspx

Limoli, Penny, *The 5 Most Common Hiring Mistakes That Are Hurting Your Practice,* http://www.dentalproductsreport.com/dental/article/5-most-common-hiring-mistakes-are-hurting-your-practice

*Hiring an Office Manager For Your Dental Practice,* http://www.warschawlearninginstitute.com/showPage.php?pg=HiringanOfficeManagerforYourDentalPractice

Ciardello, Denise, *10 Keys For Successful Hiring In Your Dental Office,* http://www.dentistryiq.com/articles/2013/10/10-keys-for-successful-hiring-in-your-dental-office.html

*The Trick To Hiring The Perfect Dental Office Manager For Your Dental Practice,* http://www.jointherevo.com/blog/the-trick-to-hiring-the-perfect-front-office-manager-for-your-dental-practice

## CHAPTER 11

*Learning Quotes,* BrainyQuote, http://www.brainyquote.com/quotes/topics/topic_learning.html

*How Do I Contribute To an Employee's Career Development,* http://

www.fsa.usda.gov/FSA/hrdapp?area=home&subject=mgrs&topic=ccd

Walter, Ekaterina, *How To Foster Employee Trust and Growth Through Constructive Feedback*, http://www.forbes.com/sites/ekaterinawalter/2013/11/19/how-to-foster-employee-trust-and-growth-through-constructive-feedback/

Llopis, Glenn, *10 Signs Your Employees Are Growing Complacent In Their Careers*, http://www.forbes.com/sites/glennllopis/2013/07/08/10-signs-your-employees-are-growing-complacent-in-their-careers/

*How Well Do Your Develop Your People?*, http://www.mindtools.com/pages/article/team-development.htm

Doyle, Alison, *How Often Do People Change Jobs?*, http://jobsearch.about.com/od/employmentinformation/f/change-jobs.htm

## CHAPTER 12

*Incentives Quotes*, BrainyQuote, http://www.brainyquote.com/quotes/keywords/incentives.html

*What About Bonus Incentives*, http://www.dentistryiq.com/articles/wdj/print/volume-3/issue-2/you-and-your-practice/what-about-bonus-incentives.html

*Team Incentive Bonus Plans*, http://www.dentaleconomics.com/articles/print/volume-98/issue-5/features/team-incentive-bonus-plans.html

*Should Your Start a Staff Incentive Program?*, http://thecuriousdentist.com/should-you-start-a-staff-incentive-program/

Anderson, Jerry, *What Are Incentive Plans?*, http://smallbusiness.chron.com/incentive-plans-1776.html

*Top 10 Reasons Why Your Company Needs an Employee Incentive Program*, http://www.incentivequotes.com/top10-reasons-why-you-employee-incentive-program.html

Dr Scott, Dow, *The Impact of Rewards Programs on Employee Engagement*, http://www.worldatwork.org/waw/adimLink?id=39032

*The Incentive Research Foundation Resource Center,* http://theirf.org/research/content/6000065/incentives-motivation-and-workplace-performance-research-and-best-practices/

## CHAPTER 13

*Communication Quotes,* BrainyQuote, http://www.brainyquote.com/quotes/topics/topic_communication.html

*Dentists Told, Brush Up On Communication Skills,* http://www.dentistry.co.uk/news/dentists-told-brush-communication-skills

*DDU Advises Dental Professional To Communicate Clearly With Patients To Comply With New Ethical Rules,* http://www.theddu.com/press-centre/press-releases/ddu-advises-dental-professionals-to-communicate-clearly-with-patients

Agarwal, Anil, *Communication Skills of Top Producing Practices,* http://www.dentaleconomics.com/articles/print/volume-101/issue-7/features/communication-skills-of-top-producing-practices.html

*Top 10 Skills For Success In Dental Communication,* http://www.ncdental.org/images/ncds/Wright%20-%20Top%2010%20Skills%20for%20Success%20in%20Dental%20Communication.pdf

Bryant, Hollie, *How to Increase Communication in Eight Areas of the Dental Office,* http://www.dentistryiq.com/articles/2011/07/how-to-increase-communication-in-eight-areas-of-the-dental-office.html

*Anyone Can Learn To Communicate Better,* https://www.protectorplan.com/wp-content/uploads/documents/benefits/risk-management/Communication.pdf

## CHAPTER 14

*Customer Quotes,* BrainyQuote, http://www.brainyquote.com/quotes/keywords/customer.html

Nation, Kristie, *Social Media – It's Just Word of Mouth Marketing,* http://www.dentaleconomics.com/articles/print/volume-103/issue-2/technology-needs/social-media-its-just-word-of-mouth-marketing.html

Sligting, Douglas, *Why Do Patient Choose You?,* http://sidekickmag.

com/continuing_education/why-do-patients-choose-you/

Lovitt, Rob, *Look Who's Talking: Patient Personas Can Provide Invaluable Insights*, http://medibeauty.biz/look-whos-talking-patient-personas-can-provide-invaluable-insights/

*23 Tips To Keep Your Patient Happy, Loyal*, http://www.dentalproductsreport.com/dental/article/23-tips-keep-your-patients-happy-loyal

*10 Proven Steps To Receive More Patients*, http://dentalpracticesolutions.com/blog/2010/02/01/10-proven-steps-to-receive-more-patients/

## CHAPTER 15

*Expectation Quotes*, BrainyQuote, http://www.brainyquote.com/quotes/keywords/expectations.html

*Managing Patient Expectations*, http://www.dental-risk.com/Portals/20/articles/Patient%20Expectations.pdf

*Manage Expectations of Patients Opting for Cosmetic Dentistry*, http://www.mddus.com/mddus/news-and-media/media-centre/september-2013/cosmetic-dentistry.aspx

Montgomery, Marc, *Predictably Meeting Patient's Expectations in Esthetic Dentistry*, http://www.oralhealthgroup.com/news/predictably-meeting-patients-expectations-in-esthetic-dentistry/1001044208/?&er=NA

*Clinical Practice Management*, http://www.dental-tribune.com/articles/specialities/practice_management/17069_patient_expectations_are_changing.html

Young, Michael, *Managing Patient Expectations*, http://www.prodentalcpd.com/UserFiles/File/Articles/Business/P513_managing_patient_expectations.pdf

## CHAPTER 16

*Online Quotes*, BrainyQuote, http://www.brainyquote.com/quotes/keywords/online.html

*Health Services Success Story Legacy Dental,* http://www.hubspot.
com/customers/legacy-dental

Duty, Shauna, *How To Win Traffic and Influence Rankings,* http://
moderndentalmarketing.com/category/content-marketing-2/

Odden, Lee, *7 Ways To Use Content For Better Online Marketing,*
http://sidekickmag.com/continuing_education/7-ways-to-use-
content-for-better-online-marketing/

Lautenslager, Al, *The Doctor – Patient Connection,* http://www.
slideshare.net/algtr17/content-marketing-for-doctors-dentists-and-
practices

Ytterberg, Kaitlyn, *Building Your Online Presence: A Checklist For
Dentists,* http://www.officite.com/articles/building-your-online-
presence-a-checklist-for-dentists/

Mosley, Michael, *How To Increase Your Online Presence,* http://www.
dentistryiq.com/articles/2012/08/how-to-increase-your-online-
presence.html

## CHAPTER 17

*Trust Quotes,* BrainyQuote, http://www.brainyquote.com/quotes/
topics/topic_trust.html

Yamalik, N, *Dentist-Patient Relationship and Quality Care 2 Trust,*
http://www.ncbi.nlm.nih.gov/pubmed/15997968

Liu, Michael, *The Dentist / Patient Relationship: The Role of Dental
Anxiety,* http://scholarship.claremont.edu/cgi/viewcontent.
cgi?article=1253&context=cmc_theses

Jacquot, Jeremy, *Trust In The Dentist-Patient Relationship: A Review,*
http://www.jyi.org/issue/trust-in-the-dentist-patient-relationship-a-
review/

Rowe, Rosemary, Calnan, Michael, *Trust Relations In Health Care –
The New Agenda,* http://eurpub.oxfordjournals.org/content/16/1/4.full

Lewicki, Roy, *Trust and Trust Building,* http://www.
beyondintractability.org/essay/trust-building

## CHAPTER 18

*Flexibility Quotes*, BrainyQuote, http://www.brainyquote.com/
quotes/keywords/flexibility.html

*Flexible Payment Options*, http://www.aldiedentist.com/payment.html

*Atlanta Dentist With Flexible Payment Plans*, http://www.
puredentalhealth.com/atlanta-dentist-flexible-payment-plans-
financing.html

*Benefits of Choosing Apex Dental Care*, http://www.apexdentalcare.
net/benefits-of-choosing-apex-dental-care/

*Finance Options*, http://www.whodoesyourteeth.com/Richmond-
Dentist-Finance-Options.asp

*The List: Top 7 Products Patients Demand*, http://www.
dentalproductsreport.com/dental/article/list-top-7-products-
patients-demand

*Paying For Dental Care*, http://www.mouthhealthy.org/en/dental-
care-concerns/paying-for-dental-care/

## CHAPTER 19

*Opportunity Quotes*, BrainyQuote, http://www.brainyquote.com/
quotes/keywords/opportunity.html

Jaccarino, Janet, *Helping The Special Needs Patient Maintain Oral
Health*, http://www.dentalcare.com/en-US/dental-education/
continuing-education/ce393/ce393.aspx?ModuleName=coursecont
ent&PartID=1&SectionID=-1

*Guideline on Management of Dental Patients With Special Health Care
Needs*, http://www.aapd.org/media/Policies_Guidelines/G_SHCN.pdf

Brocklehurst, PR, *Patient Assessment In General Dental Practice –
Risk Assessment or Clinical Monitoring?*, http://www.carifree.com/
dentists/science/documents/Patientassessmentingeneraldentalprac-
ticeriskassessmentorclinicalmonitoring.pdf

*General Guidelines For Referring Dental Patients*, http://www.ada.org/
sections/professionalresources/pdfs/referring_guidelines.pdf

Tahir, Ali, *Assessment and Investigation of Patients*, http://www.
slideshare.net/dralitahir/assessment-investigation-of-dental-
patient-12048093

Levin, Roger, *Leverage Your Most Powerful Source For New Dental
Patients*, http://www.dentistryiq.com/articles/2013/02/leverage-your-
most-powerful-source-for-new-dental-patients.html

## CHAPTER 20

Zaibak, Omar, *99 Legendary Customer Service Quotes*, http://www.
customer1.com/blog/customer-service-quotes

Fox, Karen, *Emotional Intelligence Trumps IQ In Dentist Patient
Relationship*, https://www.ada.org/news/8623.aspx

Quarantelli, Enrico, *The Dental Student Image Of The Dentist Patient
Relationship*, http://ajph.aphapublications.org/doi/pdf/10.2105/
AJPH.51.9.1312

Corah, NL, O'Shea, RM, *The Dentist-Patient Relationship: Perceptions
By Patient of Dentist Behavior in Relation To Satisfaction and Anxiety*,
http://www.ncbi.nlm.nih.gov/pubmed/3862704

*Dentistry's Dispute Resolution Program*, http://www.ada.org/sections/
professionalResources/pdfs/Peer_Review_Brochure.pdf

Rankin, JA, Harris, MB, *Patients Preference For Dentists Behaviors*,
http://www.ncbi.nlm.nih.gov/pubmed/3858344

Tse, Iris, *In Better Health: Doctor-Patient Relationships Show
Improvement*, http://www.livescience.com/13014-doctor-patient-
relationships-improving.html

# About the Author

A twenty-year dental industry veteran, Michael Hill owns a dental lab in Southern California, 6-11 Dental Studio, where he has worked with and developed solid business relationships with hundreds of dental professionals in 14 states. In that capacity, he has had the opportunity to not only observe first hand but also to gain a deep understanding of the inner workings of dental offices. He has authored three books and more than twenty-five articles on business management specifically related to the dental industry.

Hill is a regular speaker, contributor, and sponsor of educational seminars related to the successful growth and marketing of dental practices. For more information on Hill, visit **www.611dentalstudio.com**.

www.ingramcontent.com/pod-product-compliance
Lightning Source LLC
Chambersburg PA
CBHW051723170526
45167CB00002B/782